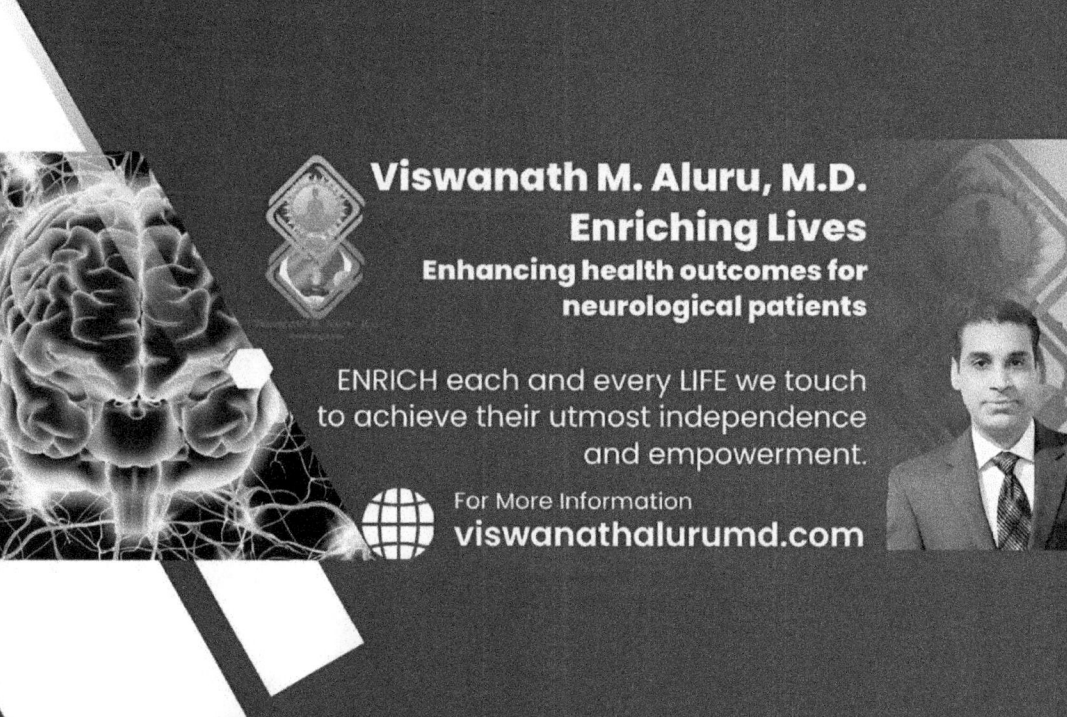

SUCCESS SERIES

PATHWAY TO U.S RESIDENCY AND MATCH

SUCCESS STRATEGIES FOR US GRADUATE MEDICAL EDUCATION, RESIDENCY APPLICATION, INTERVIEW AND MATCH

FIRST EDITION

VISWANATH M. ALURU, M.D.

Copyright by Viswanath M. Aluru, M.D.

All Rights Reserved

No part of this book may be used or reproduced in whatsoever manner without the written permission of the author.

ISBN Paper Back:979-8-9923404-3-3
ISBN Hardcover: 979-8-9923404-4-0
Library of Congress Control Number: 2025930200

I am grateful to the Almighty, my parents, brother, wife Teza, children Vedaanth and Tanvi for their everlasting and unwavering support through all these years.

I am grateful to my teachers, mentors, friends, family members, well-wishers, co-workers, colleagues, patients and their families who always stand as an inspiration to me.

About the Author

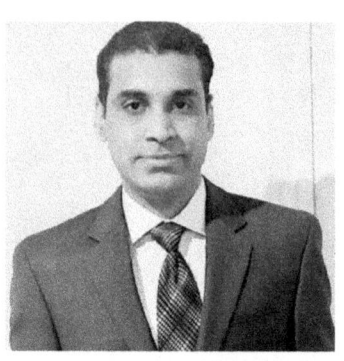

Dr. Viswanath M. Aluru, M.D. brings over 13 years of experience in enhancing health outcomes for patients with neurological disorders through compassionate care and innovative research.

With over 13 years of extensive experience as a physician and researcher, Dr. Aluru is dedicated to enhancing the quality of life and health outcomes for patients suffering from neurological disorders. As an attending physician at Ochsner Health, he specializes in delivering comprehensive care and rehabilitation for a diverse range of conditions, including stroke, brain injuries, spinal cord injuries, poly trauma and complex neurological conditions. Dr. Aluru is active in several professional organizations, including the American Academy of Physical Medicine and Rehabilitation, American Society of Neurorehabilitation, and the World Stroke Organization. Dr. Aluru's passion for patient care drives his efforts to integrate new medical advancements into practice, ensuring that those he cares for receive the highest standard of treatment.

Dr. Aluru authored several research articles, abstracts, posters in the field of Neurorehabilitation and Stroke/Brain injury rehabilitation. He presented his research at several conferences. Dr. Aluru earned his medical degree from Dr. N.T.R. University of Health Sciences, Gandhi Medical College, Secunderabad, India. He completed his internship training in General Surgery at University of Illinois, Chicago and residency training in Physical Medicine and Rehabilitation at Kingsbrook Jewish Medical Center, One Brooklyn Health System, Brooklyn, NY.

He is always at the forefront of teaching medical students and residents. He participates in inpatient teaching rounds, journal clubs, grand rounds with the medical students and residents. He also serves as a mentor for medical students and residents in research projects.

Disclaimer

USMLE is a registered trademark and is jointly organized by Federation of State Medical Boards (FSMB) and National Board of Medical Examiners (NBME). FREIDA is a registered trademark of American Medical Association (AMA). Terms NRMP, MATCH, SOAP, FindAResident are registered trademarks of American Association of Medical Colleges (AAMC). ECFMG is a trademark of Intealth. The author does not own or claim any of these terms. They are only used in connection with the chapters in the book.

PREFACE

I am excited to bring this book US Residency and Match for US graduate medical residency program aspiring applicants. Several of you have contacted me for guidance with the application process, interview preparation and residency match. It's a big topic. I wanted to focus on important points in each chapter of this book. First, congratulations to all of you because you worked hard through all these years. You've come a long way and now you're at the crucial step to gain your foot into a residency program. This step is crucial because now you really must showcase your hard work through all these years in the process of your residency application. In this book, I will start with a brief note on US health care system and how residency programs work. Thereafter, I will take your through the residency journey starting with preparation for USMLE, creating your ERAS token and account, residency program search process, sorting through the programs, preparing your application documents, uploading documents to your ERAS account, submitting your ERAS application, preparing for the interview, how to ace your interview, preparing your rank order list, creating your NRMP account, submitting rank order list, MATCH day, post-MATCH process including supplemental offer program, applying for off cycle positions. I hope this book with serve as your companion as you navigate through this complex process. Should you have any further questions or needing any further advice, feel free to send me an e-mail to Viswanath.Aluru@gmail.com. I would be happy to answer your questions. With this let's jump right into Pathway to US Residency and Match. All the very best in finding your top choice program.

Acknowledgements

I am excited to bring this book to all the aspiring US graduate medical training applicants. I want to thank my faculty, senior friends, my classmates from my medical school who gave me advice and support when I wanted to pursue US residency training. I also want to thank Kaplan Medical, USMLE World, Dr. Red Archer CCS training for being my USMLE training partners. My sincere thanks to Dr. Farooq, Houston, TX for allowing me to observe him while rounding through various hospitals in Texas Medical Center. I want to thank Dr. Green at Moffitt Cancer Center, USF Health, Tampa, FL for giving me an opportunity in their International Vising Scholars Program which provided me invaluable experience. I want to thank Dr. Richter, Emory Medical Center, Atlanta, GA; Dr. Phillips, Atlanta Medical Center, Atlanta, GA for allowing me to rotate as a sub-intern. I am grateful for their valuable advice and mentoring.

My interest in the field of Physical Medicine and Rehabilitation and Neurorehabilitation stemmed from working as a volunteer in the Motor Recovery Lab at department of PM&R, Rusk Institute of Rehabilitation Medicine, New York University Grossman School of Medicine, New York, USA. I am forever grateful to my mentor Dr. Preeti Raghavan who accepted me as a volunteer in her research lab then as a research associate, assistant research scientist working on several projects involving stroke, brain injury population which strengthened my knowledge and understanding of the field. This position allowed me to present and publish several abstracts, research articles, posters that provided invaluable knowledge, experience further enhancing my CV. I am grateful to Dr. Cohen, Dr. Ahn, Dr. Flanagan and Dr. Moroz in the PM&R department at NYU Rusk Rehabilitation for allowing me to follow them in their morning rounds, clinics to gain hands on clinical experience, letters of recommendation that boosted my confidence and strengthened my residency application. I am forever grateful to the UIC General

Surgery Associate Program Director Dr. Havelka who called me for an interview when I was eagerly looking to find my internship spot. I fondly cherished my training and mentorship with General Surgery residency (internship) training at UIC Chicago with chairman Dr. Benedetti and residency program director Dr. Borhani and all the department faculty, staff and my co-residents and fellows. My sincere thanks to chairman of my PM&R residency training program at Kingsbrook Jewish Medical Center, Brooklyn, NY Dr. Ross, program director Dr. Christian who gave me an opportunity for an interview and had immense confidence in my abilities as a resident physician. I am also thankful to my other PM&R residency program directors throughout the training Dr. Lefkowitz, Dr. Dinescu, rest of PM&R faculty, staff, co-residents for their valuable education, mentoring, support throughout the training.

I am grateful to Dr. Karlin, chairman of department of Physical Medicine and Rehabilitation at Ochsner Clinic Foundation, Ochsner Health, New Orleans, LA, USA for offering me first full-time position as an inpatient PM&R physician right after my residency graduation amidst pandemic.

I am greatly indebted to my parents Siromani Sarma and Rama Devi Aluru who instilled in me great values and upbringing. My love and gratitude to my brother Phani Krishna Aluru for his support throughout my childhood, schooling, college and medical school. I would not be writing this today without unconditional support from my wife Teza Aluru through all ups and downs, throughout my internship and residency training, early career post training taking care of our children. I am grateful to my close friends and family who always stood as pillars of strength through tough times and good times. My unending love to my children Vedaanth and Tanvi Aluru who always bring so much joy, energy and enthusiasm.

I want to thank our publishers McMillan Publishing, Miami, FL for helping me from time to time with all aspects from drafting, proof reading, editing, design, publishing, marketing. I want to thank Amazon and other platforms for their support with marketing, sales.

Viswanath M. Aluru, M.D.
New Orleans, LA, USA.
www.viswanathalurumd.com

Content

Chapter 1: US Health Care System and Residency Training 1

Chapter 2: USMLE performance and residency 5

Chapter 3: Residency program search and selection 9

Chapter 4: ERAS application 17

Chapter 5: Interview Selection Process 29

Chapter 6: Interview preparation and interview 36

Chapter 7: Rank order list 45

Chapter 8: NRMP MATCH 52

Chapter 9: Supplemental MATCH and off cycle positions 55

Chapter 10: Visa Requirements for IMGs 58

Chapter 11: Not matched, now what? 63

Chapter 12: Final remarks 65

    APPENDIX A 67

    APPENDIX B 70

    APPENDIX C 79

    APPENDIX Di 100

    APPENDIX Dii 127

    APPENDIX Diii 136

GLOSSARY 150

INDEX 151

NOTES 153

Chapter 1: US Health Care System and Residency Training

a. US Health care system

You might be wondering sometimes if this residency process takes too long; it may or may not happen. You might also think that it's not a fair process for all the candidates.

I want to tell you why you must go through so much of this process, starting with the USMLE and then going through the application process, interview, rank order list, and match.

The reason is there's a lot of liability involved with the healthcare in this country. For the chairman of a department, the goal is to keep the department as number one in the country or in the top position in the country, to attract top talent, top faculty, and to attract top research dollars or funding for the department. For a program director, because the residency programs run entirely on taxpayer dollars or Medicare dollars, they want to make sure that they attract good candidates who can complete their residency training in good standing. The program director also wants to make sure residents can complete the yearly exams and board exams so that they don't lose accreditation status or lose good standing for the residency program.

For attending physicians, because residents work directly under attending physicians, they must endorse every document that residents enter in the medical records. They want to make sure that the patients are getting appropriate treatment and ongoing communication regarding what's going on with their health and that they're taken care of properly in a timely manner. Attending physicians also must ensure that the documentation is taken care of on time.

For hospital management, they must make sure that the hospitals don't get penalized or that there is no problem for their license for the hospitals. There's a lot of scrutiny involved. That's the reason why residency applicants must go through so many steps to make sure that they are able to do the job appropriately and complete their residency training on time. That's one way of looking at it. The other way is that all these USMLE scores represent something. USMLE Step 1 represents basic science knowledge, and Step 2 CK represents the ability to apply clinical knowledge to clinical skills. USMLE Step 3 represents actual training ability to take care of the patients in a real-time setting. Passing USMLE exams with good scores on the first attempt also represents the applicant's ability or performance on the yearly tests in the residency training and performance in the specialty board exam after the training. That's why the program directors rely too much on these board scores or standardized test scores. They also want to see the applicant's performance in the clerkships and the letters of recommendation from physicians or specialists because that's going to tell how they are going to perform in the residency training rotations as well. This sums up why this entire process is too long. When it comes to interviews, it is the most important criterion that can make or break any residency application because programs want to know the candidate in person at a very personal level to know about their personality, attitude, ability to carry along with other people in the training, communication strategies, time management, and so on. For these reasons, the interview is one of the most important criteria.

At the end of the day, we all want to make sure that we are giving the best possible training. We want to make sure that trainees are getting the best out of every residency program in a very safe environment.

Vis Tip: Once you have an interview, your goal should be to ace your interview irrespective of any red flags or gaps in your application.

b. Residency positions and number of applicants:

Let me give you an example of how the residency interview and selection process go. Say, for example, a program that you are applying to has five spots for this year, and they received 5 thousand applications for five spots. That means 1000 applications for each spot. Now each residency program has its own filtration criteria. That's the only way they can get through all these applications because they are not even going to look at all these applications. The programs set their filters. Based on their filters, let's assume the program filtered out all the candidates and selected 500 candidates from that 5 thousand pool of applications. That means for each spot, the program has selected 100 applicants. From those 500 applications, the residency selection committee, let's say, selected 100 applicants for interviews. Which means that the program is inviting 20 candidates for interviews for each spot. Out of these 100 applicants at the interview, they will apply some ranking system, and then the program, let's say, will submit a rank order list for the top 30 candidates. That means for five spots, imagine that the program is submitting a rank order list for the top 30 candidates. Which means that for each spot, the program ranked six candidates.

If the candidate is in the top ten or maybe top 15, the chances of getting matched into that program are high. That is the level of competition for US graduate medical residency programs.

Key Points:

- Residency application is a lengthy process.
- Board scores, clerkship scores, and personalized letters of recommendation play a crucial role.

- *Being in top 10 or top 15 of the program's rank list greatly increases chance of matching into a program.*
- *The interview is the most important step in the final selection process.*

Chapter 2: USMLE performance and residency

a. USMLE exams and recent changes:

USMLE comprises step one, step two, and step three exams. When I took the exams, there was a three-digit score and a two-digit score on each step. However, with recent changes, USMLE Step 1 is no longer a three-digit or two-digit score. It's a pass or fail system. USMLE Step 2 still has a three-digit score for the CK component (clinical knowledge), but it no longer has a clinical skills (CS) exam. That means it's only step 2 CK. There is no longer a USMLE Step 2 CS. USMLE Step 3 comprises part one and part two. Based on your performance on step 3, part one and part two, you will get a three-digit and a two-digit score.

b. USMLE step 1 new scoring system:

Because USMLE Step 1 is a pass or fail system, you really must work hard to get a pass on the first attempt. Because of this new scoring system on step 1, programs can't gauge your application. The applicant is at a disadvantage because, if you have a three-digit scoring system on step 1, then based on that three-digit score, the program can look at the rest of your application to estimate your performance. However, if it is simply a pass or fail system, if you fail on the first attempt, they might not even look at your application. That's why the applicants are at a disadvantage from my personal point of view.

c. USMLE step 2 CK score is the key:

USMLE Step 2 CK has a three-digit scoring system. Every program has its own set criteria. Some programs require at least a 220 three-digit score on step 2 CK. It is important for you to get a first attempt pass on USMLE Step 1 and a good score on USMLE Step 2 to be at a competitive advantage.

d. When do you need to complete USMLE step 3?

Some candidates might want to consider USMLE Step 3. Ideally you don't need a step three score to apply to a residency program. For international medical graduates (IMGs), once you have obtained an ECFMG certificate (after completion of USMLE step 1 and 2), you are eligible to apply for the USMLE step 3 exam. Every residency program has its own rules for USMLE Step 3 completion. Some programs require it by the end of the first year of residency or the second year, but before graduating from the residency program, you need to have a step three score. It becomes difficult to focus on step three preparation once you start your residency training. I recommend that if you have time between interviews and before starting your residency year, you try to complete the exam so you don't have to worry about it when you're busy in your residency training.

e. Types of residency program applicants:

There are two types of residency applicants.

- US Graduates.
- International Medical Graduates (IMGs).

International medical graduates are further classified as truly international medical graduates who graduated and completed all their clinical rotations from an international medical school. There are certain international medical schools where they complete their basic sciences and clinical skills and then come to the United States to complete their clinical rotations. They are a different category of the international medical graduates. Even though they are considered international medical graduates, they are at a greater advantage compared to truly international graduates.

f. Is USMLE step 3 needed for applying:

If you're an international medical graduate and if your performance on USMLE Step 2 is in the moderate range, then you might want to consider having a Step 3 score before the interview season or at least before submitting your rank order list. Keep in mind that step 3 is a highly clinical exam that has part 1 and part 2 CCS. If you haven't started your residency training, you may find it difficult to take this test. Unless you're confident that you're going to pass this exam, you must prepare well before attempting it. You don't want to have a negative score on the step three exam before the interview season or before the ranking list. The programs will know once you have completed the exam or once you have a score on the exam. If you are not confident enough to take the test, then submitting your application with USMLE step one and step 2 results would be a better option.

Vis Tip: *If you are an international medical graduate, having a step three score will boost your application.*

g. USMLE resources:

I want you all to be familiar with the USMLE website, www.usmle.org, which has several resources that you can download. It will give you strategies for preparation. You can also download the USMLE simulation software and practice questions. On the same website, you can also apply for USMLE step one, step two, and step three examinations as well.

There's another website—NBME (National Board of Medical Examiners)—where you can do a mock test that almost resembles a USMLE test. I recommend you take this NBME mock exam a month before your actual USMLE exam. It gives you a summary of your results and the areas that you need to focus on before you take the actual USMLE exam.

h. ECFMG certificate:

This is important for International Medical Graduates, or IMGs. Once you have your USMLE Step 1 and Step 2 score results, go to the ECFMG—Educational Commission for Foreign Medical Graduates—website and apply for an ECFMG certificate. ECFMG will issue a certificate stating that you have fulfilled all the requirements for USMLE step one and step two.

When you are applying for an ACGME-accredited residency program, if you don't upload your ECFMG certificate as an IMG, your application won't even be considered for a review. It might take up to four to six weeks for you to receive the physical copy of your ECFMG certificate by mail. Plan to apply for the certificate early before the start of the residency application season.

Key points:

- *Have a pass on the first attempt on step one.*
- *Get a good score on step two, at least 220.*
- *If you have more than one attempt on step one, then aim for a higher score on step two, at least 240 score, to be competitive.*
- *IMGs will be at a greater advantage when competing with the US medical graduates by having a USMLE Step 3 score.*

Chapter 3: Residency program search and selection

I request you all to take this information as general advice. Each specialty is different, and each residency program is different; they have their own criteria.

a. How do you search for residency programs?

One important website I want you all to be familiar with is the American Medical Association (AMA) FREIDA Online. It's a great resource for residency applicants. It has all the resources that are free of cost. You have the option to access in-depth content at some fee. You can search their entire database by specialty, state, and several other criteria.

b. When to start searching for residency programs?

I highly recommend you start this residency program search process in mid-June. Spend about one or two hours every day. Create a spreadsheet by your specialty for each state.

List all requirements for each program:

- How many attempts on the exam?
- What are the USMLE step score requirements?
- How many years from the date of graduation?
- How many letters of recommendation?
- What types of clinical rotations are there, and for how long?
- US clinical experience and for how long?
- Do they accept IMGs?
- Do they require an ECFMG certificate?
- Do they offer visas, and what type of visas do they offer?
- What is the step 3 requirement?
- Do they need any research experience?

These are some of the important criteria you must include in your program spreadsheet. Be ready with the programs list that you want to apply to at least by mid-August. In that way, you are ready to apply to those programs when the ERAS application opens in September.

c. Know the difference between ERAS season and ERAS application time:

It's important to know that each year, ERAS season opens in mid-June. That's when you get your ERAS token and register with AAMC to get your AAMC ID and activate your ERAS account.

The ERAS application opens in September. That's when you submit your application to all the desired programs.

You should start working on your residency application (supporting documents, including contacting letter writers), searching for programs starting in June, not in August or in September.

Vis Tip: *Be ready to submit your application on the day that the ERAS application opens!*

d. Beware of consultants and brokers!

Let me tell you that several agencies or consultants will lure you with the promise that they're going to place you in the residency programs and will put you in direct contact with the program directors. Please do not listen to these people. They will charge you thousands of dollars. The truth is no one is going to place you in any residency program. Even if you know someone in a residency program, the maximum they can do for you is get your application in front of the program director if they haven't already reviewed your application. You must go through the residency application process. National Residency Match Program (NRMP) or some other match program unless that program is not participating in the match. That's the only way you can get into a residency program.

e. Do I need to apply to several programs?

There is a misconception among applicants that by applying to several programs, their chances of matching will increase. That's not true. If your residency application does not meet the program requirements, they are not even going to look at your application. I highly recommend you do your homework. You prepare your program list by mid-August and apply to those programs selectively that will increase your chances of interviews and thereby increase your chances of getting into a residency program.

Vis Tip: Apply only to those programs that you meet their criteria

f. Types of residency programs and requirements:

There are four different types of residency programs:

University programs in university hospitals

University-affiliated programs—these are hospitals that have some kind of affiliation with the university.

Community programs these are smaller hospitals in the community.

Rural track programs or rural programs in the rural areas.

Each type of program has different requirements. Obviously, university programs require higher USMLE scores compared to university-affiliated, community hospitals or rural programs.

g. Do I need high 260 scores on step 2 and step 3?

Don't be under the impression that you need to have 240 or 260 scores on USMLE Step 2 CK and Step 3 to apply to residency programs. Even if you have moderate scores like in the 200-210 range, you are eligible to apply to the residency program. That's why it's important that you do your homework depending on your scores, depending on your clinical experience, letters of recommendation, and other criteria. Select only those programs that you can apply to that will increase your chances of getting a residency interview and eventually getting into the residency program.

Residency checklist:

- Prepare for USMLE step one and step two.
- Take the NBME mock test before the final exam.
- Apply for an ECFMG certificate if you are an international medical graduate.
- Reach out to your letter writers in mid-June.
- Start your residency program search process in June.
- Prepare your list of the programs based on your criteria.
- Be ready with the program list by the time the ERAS application opens in September.
- Don't fall prey to consultants or brokers.

h. **Important websites to remember:**

www.usmle.org – For USMLE prep and USMLE exam scheduling

www.nbme.org – For mock test and prep

www.ecfmg.org – For ECFMG certificate, applicant tracking system, SEVIS (J1), ERAS token

https://freida.ama-assn.org – American Medical Association FREIDA online residency program directory.

www.aamc.org - Association of American Medical Colleges

www.myeras.aamc.org - Electronic Residency Application Service (ERAS)

www.nrmp.org – National Residency Match Program

These are the most important websites to remember throughout your residency application process and match process. There is also a lot of information on the residency program websites that you want to apply to.

i. Can I contact the program before application?

If you don't find some information that you need to decide whether you want to apply to that program, you can directly contact the program director or program coordinator. I highly recommend you do so during the early months like June or July, but not towards the end of August or September when the residency season is already starting. The programs receive thousands of emails, so they won't be able to respond to your email. Please contact them early if you need any additional information.

j. Where else I can find my specialty-specific information?

There are specialty-specific websites, for example, AMA or AAFP for Family Medicine, AAP for Pediatrics, AAPM&R for Physical Medicine and Rehabilitation, AAN for Neurology, ACS for General Surgery, and so on. The specialty-specific websites also have a wealth of information and resources for medical students and aspiring residents. Please look at those websites.

k. Tag team!

Residency program search is a tedious process. Thankfully with an online program directory and specialty-specific websites, you would be able to search programs by various criteria and be able to save the list and your search criteria. I recommend if you have any friends who are applying to the same specialty, tag team, divide, and conquer. In that way, it doesn't take too much time for just one person doing everything.

I. **Types of residency programs:**
- It is important to know the various types of residency programs.
- There are mainly three types of residency programs.
- Preliminary or transitional year program, which is a year program
- Categorical program—where you can complete your entire residency training in just one program.
- Advanced program—which does not offer internship training, however, offers advanced specialty training

Categorical programs:

Categorical programs are either three-year, four-year programs, or even five-to-seven-year programs, depending on the specialty. For example, Internal Medicine, Family Medicine, and Pediatrics are all three-year categorical programs. Physical Medicine and Rehabilitation, Neurology, and Radiology are four-year programs, and all the surgical specialties are anywhere between five to seven-year programs.

Advanced programs:

These programs do not offer internships or first-year training. You must complete the first-year internship in some other residency program or in another department in the same hospital, and then you move on to specialty training in the subsequent years. However, some programs might offer first-year or internship training in the same program. For example, Physical Medicine and Rehabilitation is a four-year program. However, not all the programs offer four years of training. They only offer second-, third-, and fourth-year training. That means you must apply to some other program to fulfill your requirement for the preliminary year or internship year, either in the same hospital or in a different hospital in the same city or an entirely different state.

It's important to know which is a categorical program and which is an advanced program so that you can decide where you want to apply depending on that information. You should create two separate spreadsheets, one for categorical programs and one for preliminary programs, and be ready with the programs that you want to apply to by the time the ERAS application opens.

m. Can I apply to multiple specialties?

It's important not to apply to multiple specialties in the same program or hospital. For example, please do not apply to Internal Medicine, Family Medicine, and Pediatrics in the same hospital. It's not advisable because somehow, they can come to know that you are applying to multiple specialties in the same program. It doesn't look good on your application. It shows that you are undecided about which specialty you want to go into. I highly recommend you apply to one specialty in one hospital unless you are applying to a four-year program, but they don't have internship training. In that situation, you can apply to a preliminary program in the same hospital.

Vis Tip: *Do not apply to multiple specialties in the same hospital.*

Key points:

- *Know the difference between ERAS season and ERAS application start dates.*
- *Do your research and have a final desired program list to apply*
- *Know the difference between different types of residency programs.*
- *Apply only to programs that match your application criteria.*

- *Apply on the day when the ERAS application opens.*
- *Do not apply to multiple specialties in the same program unless you are applying to advanced and preliminary programs.*

Chapter 4: ERAS application

ERAS is an electronic residency application service that was developed by the American Association of Medical Colleges (AAMC). I advise all the US and international residency aspirants to familiarize themselves with this website. Please go to aamc.org and go to the medical student and resident section. You have tons of resources, webinars, and videos. It's a great resource.

AAMC account

The first step is to create an account on the AAMC website. Once you create an account, it will assign you an ID, the AAMC ID, which is your identifier for the rest of the residency season, and you can also use the same AAMC ID for the following season if you wish to reapply.

My ERAS account:

Once you have your AAMC account created, then you need to open an ERAS account. If you are a US graduate, you need to request an ERAS token from your dean's office. If you're an International Medical Graduate, or IMG, you will request this token from your ECFMG account. ECFMG acts as your dean's office. The ERAS token is a one-time code that you will use to activate your AAMC account. Once you enter your ERAS token, it will give access to your ERAS account.

Difference between ERAS season and residency application season:

The ERAS season opens in June, sometime in the first week of June, whereas the residency application season opens in September. Especially it is important for international medical graduates who are not aware of this application process. If you start working on your application late at the end of August or in September, then everything will be delayed. I highly recommend starting your application preparation in June.

Open your AAMC account in June, and when the ERAS season opens in June, you request your ERAS token and enter that information in your AAMC, and that will give you access to my ERAS account.

My ERAS account:

My ERAS has four components:

ERAS profile

ERAS Application

Document section and

Residency Program section

My ERAS profile

My ERAS profile is where you update your contact information. I highly recommend you keep this information up to date because the programs see this information when they open your application.

For example, if you live in California and apply to some program in Alaska or Minnesota, the program wants to know whether you can accept this offer and be able to go to the residency program there. It's important that you keep this information up to date. When you move to different locations, please go into the ERAS profile and update your information.

ERAS application:

The next section is the ERAS application. It is a crucial step for you in your transition from being a medical graduate to a resident physician. You must showcase your hard work through all these years. That's why this ERAS application is a crucial document for you to showcase all the curricular and extracurricular activities. You can download a template of this ERAS application (see Appendix B) from the AAMC website. I highly recommend you work offline on this template. It's almost a 23-page document, so it does include all the information that you need from your undergraduate training to your medical school, clerkships, sub-internships, research experience, volunteer experience, hobbies, interests, publications, book chapters, medical society memberships, and so on. You must start this process in June. Work on this document thoroughly offline, and then once you're ready, you input that information into your ERAS application and save this document several times. You can go back to this document and edit it as many times as you want. You really want to take a thorough look at this document before you sign this document. Once you sign this document, you are not going to go back and make any changes to this document. The ERAS application is important information that goes to the programs when you apply to programs during the residency application.

i. **ERAS documents:**

The next component of my ERAS is the document section. There are several documents that you need to upload under this section. (see appendix B).

- A professional up-to-date photograph is important for the programs to see you.
- Personal statement (s)
- USMLE transcript
- ECFMG certificate (IMGs)
- Dean's Letter or Medical Student Performance Evaluation (MSPE)

- Letters of recommendations
- Medical School transcript

1. **MSPE or dean's letter:**

The Medical Student Performance Evaluation (MSPE), or Dean's letter, will be sent by your dean's office. If you're an international medical graduate, you might want to work with your medical school to get this document. Dean's letter is a summary of all your experience during medical school. Your academic performance, clinical rotations, extracurricular activities, and so on. The document will be sent to the ERAS. If you're an IMG, you can get this document uploaded directly under MY ERAS documents. The programs cannot see this document until after November, but you can still attach this document to your ERAS application to the program that you want to apply to. When the application season opens, the program will be able to download this document after November.

2. **Personal Statement:**

A personal statement is something that tells your story.

What not to include in your personal statement?

Residency program attending physicians or program directors don't want to know why you went to medical school, how much you struggled to get through the USMLE exams, or why you have more than one attempt on USMLE exams. You don't have to mention all those things at all.

What to include on your personal statement!

The residency program wants to know about your success story that shaped you into the person you are today. They want to know your qualities, your qualifications, and how you're going to fit into their program.

Remember that the residency training is anywhere between three to four years, sometimes even seven years, depending on the specialty. It's a long journey. Residency program leadership wants to know that you're going to successfully complete the program and be able to make a positive impact on it. They also want to know how you're going to contribute to this field or specialty that you have chosen to apply to. These are the things that you must include in your personal statement.

Yes, you can include some of the medical school or clinical experiences that helped you choose your specialty.

You work offline and edit it several times. Send it to people that you know are going to give you good feedback about your personal statement before you upload it to the document section.

Do I need multiple personal statements?

If you're applying to preliminary and advanced programs or different specialties, you might want to personalize your personal statement to that specialty. For example, if you're applying to Physical Medicine and Rehabilitation, but you need to also apply to a preliminary program, for example, preliminary General Surgery. Please don't send the same personal statement to both programs. You must personalize to the type of program (preliminary vs. advanced vs. categorical) and to the specialty (PM&R vs. surgery vs. medicine, and so on).

Save different personal statements with naming or identification (only you can see those file names) and attach appropriate personal statements to that program.

3. Letters of recommendation:

You must start asking your letter writers to write a letter for you in June because remember the attending physicians and program directors are busy. They have less time to focus on these letters. Please don't get disappointed if those letters don't go to ERAS on time or don't get uploaded on time if you have not contacted them early. If you contact them at the end of August or in September, they won't be able to get the letters that you need in time. It's important that you contact your letter writers early.

What to include in your email to your letter writers?

When you contact your letter writers by email, please write a summary of who you are and what you're doing right now. Attach your latest CV and a personal statement.

In that way, they know exactly what to write to make a letter of recommendation more personalized. Otherwise, they're just going to send a generic letter like anyone else; it's important to make it more personal. You must send them as much information as possible and as early as possible, in June, so they can send your letter to ERAS on time.

Whom should you contact to write your letter of recommendation?

It is important that you identify your letter writers carefully. You will know when you're doing your sub-internships or your clerkships. You will understand who those attendings or program directors are that you want to approach for a letter. The key to getting an outstanding letter of recommendation is that they need to know you and understand you on a personal level.

Whether to waive or not to waive your right to see the letter?

You could either request the letter to be given to you directly or request to send the letters to the ERAS. It works in both ways. If the letter writer sends your letter directly to ERAS, you are waiving your right to see the letter of recommendation.

On the other side, once your letter writers hand over the letter to you, you could scan the letters and upload them into the letters of recommendation section on the ERAS account.

How to assign letters to letter writers on ERAS?

Create an empty slot with the letter writer's name and upload the scanned document. For those letters that you waived (going directly to the ERAS), you still must create an empty slot with the letter writer's name on the ERAS account. When the letter writer sends your letter to the ERAS directly, ERAS will scan the letter for you and upload it into your document folder also known as ERAS Post Office.

For example, letters A and B have already been uploaded to the ERAS account. For letters C and D, you waived your right to see those letters. However, you created empty slots with the letter writers' names on your ERAS account.

How to choose appropriate letters of recommendation:

Let's review an example. If you are applying to the Physical Medicine and Rehabilitation residency program. You want to apply to an advanced PM&R program for second, third and 4th year training. However, you also need an internship program for first year training. Depending on the type of program or the specialty you're applying to, you must choose letters of recommendation appropriately. You could attach up to four letters of recommendation. I recommend you attach at least two letters related to the primary specialty. In this example, your primary specialty is Physical Medicine and Rehabilitation. In case, you don't have any primary specialty letters from the letter writers, you could upload the letters that are available. I highly recommend you have at least one letter from the primary specialty. In this example, if you're applying to a Physical Medicine and Rehabilitation residency program and an Internal Medicine internship program. You might want to select two Physical Medicine and Rehabilitation letters of recommendation and two Internal Medicine letters of recommendation. In that way, it's balanced. However, the mix of letters of recommendation could vary depending on what is available to you as a candidate.

What if I don't have any US letters of recommendation:

International Medical graduates (IMGs), who complete and graduate from their medical school in a foreign country, may not have any US clinical experience or could obtain any US physician letters of recommendation. That is totally acceptable. They could request letters from their medical school and hospital faculty or any other attendings or faculty outside the medical school that they worked with after medical school training.

How do programs access your letters of recommendation (waived vs un-waived letters)?

In your ERAS application, you must check the boxes next to those letters that you want to send to the programs. When you submit your application, the program will be able to see what letters of recommendation you have submitted.

Once the waived letters are uploaded to the ERAS post office, the programs that you are applying to will be able to download the letters directly from the ERAS Post Office. However, you must check the boxes for those letters in your ERAS application while applying to programs, so that they can access the letters from the ERAS Post Office.

For un waived letters, you could directly upload the letters to your ERAS account and select by checking the boxes on the application.

Once you submit your application, programs will be able to download those letters directly along with your ERAS application.

ii. Residency program selection list on ERAS:

By this time, you might have already created spreadsheets related to which programs you want to apply.

Let's consider an example specialty: Physical Medicine and Rehabilitation residency. Let's imagine that you want to apply to 50 PM&R programs. Out of these 50 PM&R residency programs, let's assume 10 programs are categorical—that means they offer a four-year training. The rest of the 40 programs are advanced, which means they only offer second, third, and 4th-year residency training.

When you apply to advanced training programs, you must apply to first-year internship programs as well. Let's say you selected 100 programs for internships. Out of these 100 programs, 50 are internal medicine internship programs and 50 are general surgery preliminary training programs. The total program count is 150, out of which 50 programs are your primary specialty, which is Physical Medicine and Rehabilitation, and 100 programs are for internship training. Out of these 100 internship programs, 50 are for internal medicine and 50 are for preliminary surgery.

In your ERAS account, you need to search for the programs that you want to apply to, and you must save them under your ERAS account. In the above example, you would search for all these 150 programs and save them under your ERAS account.

Don't forget to attach supporting documents!

There's one last step that is remaining before the application season opens. Once you have saved all the 150 programs, open each saved program, check the boxes next to the supporting documents, and save again. Once you open the program that you saved, it will show you all the supporting documents that you have attached to your application.

   a. **ERAS documents checklist:**
   - Please also refer to Appendix B.
   - Profile photo
   - Up-to-date CV
   - ERAS application
   - Letters of recommendation
   - Personal statement
   - Dean's letter or medical student performance evaluation.
   - Medical school transcript
   - USMLE transcript
   - ECFMG certificate (IMGs)

These are the main supporting documents. Depending on which boxes you're checking, only those supporting documents will be transmitted to the program when you submit your application. Keep in mind some of the documents are directly transmitted by ERAS to the program once you check the appropriate box. By default, once you apply to a program, the program will be able to see and download your ERAS application, but the rest of the supporting documents depend on which ones you are selecting. When the application season opens in September, all you do is hit the submit button!

   b. **The residency application process is expensive!**

You must know that applying to residency programs is expensive. Please refer to the AAMC website for the latest information on the pricing. For the first 10 or 11 programs, it will cost you maybe $25-$30. After that, each program will cost you around 30 dollars. You must estimate how much it's going to cost you if you need to apply to 150 programs (in the above example) so you can plan accordingly.

Please have that amount available when the application season opens so that you don't have to wait for anything.

Please refer to Appendix B for the ERAS checklist.

c. Applying to non-ERAS programs:

If you don't find a certain program that you want to apply to, that means that the program may not be participating in the Electronic Residence Application Service (ERAS). You might want to contact the program directly to know how the program wants to transmit your application and supporting documents. They might have their own application process. Most of the programs and specialties participate in ERAS. However, some programs may not participate in ERAS; they might stay as a non-ERAS program.

Key points:

Request an ERAS token from the dean's office or ECFMG (IMGs).

- *Create an AAMC account and activate My ERAS using the ERAS token.*
- *Request letters of recommendation from letter writers.*
- *Start searching for programs in your desired specialty.*
- *My ERAS account document checklist*
- *Professional photograph*
- *Personal statement/s*
- *Letters of recommendation (non-waived)*
- *Medical Student Performance Evaluation (MSPE)*
- *ECFMG certificate (IMGs)*
- *Medical school transcript*
- *USMLE or COMLEX transcript*

Save programs under your My ERAS account and attach appropriate documents.

Apply to the program when the ERAS application opens.

Chapter 5: Interview Selection Process

Once you submit the ERAS application, I highly advise you not to contact programs immediately either by email or phone. Each program receives thousands of emails and applications. They may not be able to personally respond to every application candidate or every request. Please maintain patience, as every program has its own timelines as to when they are going to review these applications and when they will start the interview process.

Applicant Document Tracking System (ADTS):

Once you log in to your ERAS account, you will see the ADTS Application Document Tracking System. ADTS tells you which programs you applied to, which programs downloaded your application, and what supporting documents were downloaded. You will know where in the process your application is.

In that way, you can have some information regarding your application download and review status.

Vis Tip: Please maintain patience while waiting.

Will I receive a confirmation?

Please don't take things personally if you don't hear from the program because it's not just you. Most of the candidates may not hear from the programs because of the number of applications they're receiving. Some programs might send you a receipt notice or a refusal notice, but some programs may not communicate with you at all. If you don't meet their selection criteria, you may not hear from that program. That's important to keep in mind.

a. Peak interview season:

The peak interview season goes from anywhere between October through the end of January. Sometimes interviews can go into the first week of February but not afterwards because the programs mainly want to focus on preparing their rank order list and submit their final rank order list by the last week of February.

Be mindful of the holiday season, like Thanksgiving, Christmas, and New Year holidays. You may not have any interviews during those holidays and a few days before and after. Please make sure to schedule your interviews for the season, keeping in mind those holidays.

When do you hear from the program after submitting an application?

Once you submit your application, if you don't hear from the program even after the end of October, if you qualify for their interview criteria, then you should try to call the program or send an email to the coordinator saying that you're interested in the program and looking forward to having an interview. I do not recommend you walk into a program if you're in the same city because that might go in the opposite direction for you.

Delayed or incomplete application:

As early as possible, once the ERAS application season opens, you must submit your complete application. If you submit your application and delay sending the supporting documents or do not send all the supporting documents, then the program may not be able to decide whether to give you an interview based on the incomplete application.

Vis Tip: *Submit as soon as possible and submit a complete application. Only then your chances of getting an interview in that program will improve.*

b. Supporting documents weightage:

1. Medical school Performance:

The medical school transcript will give the program director or attending some information about your performance in the medical school.

2. Clerkship performance:

One of the most important selection criteria is your clerkship performance. If you're an international medical graduate and if you don't have US clinical experience, I recommend that you either do a clerkship before graduation from the International Medical School or after graduation. If you're in the US on some visa, try to find a sub-internship or externship program. It is challenging for international medical graduates to get into a sub-internship or externship program. You might have to contact the Clerkship Office or Medical Student Education Office to find out if they have any clerkships or sub-internships available for international graduates and what the process is.

Having hands-on clinical experience carries enormous weight in terms of your application selection for the interview.

What if I am unable to do a clerkship?

If you are unable to get a sub-internship or externship or any hands-on clinical experience in the US (especially for foreign medical students), at least try to do observership or shadowing, which might carry some weightage but not that much compared to a hands-on clinical experience. It is not only about experience, but it will also put you in direct contact with the attending physician or whoever you are working with, and you will be able to get a strong personalized letter of recommendation after you complete your rotation.

3. USMLE performance:

Remember, USMLE scores carry significant weight in deciding whether you will receive an interview call or not. Having said that, I want to advise you all that USMLE scores are not the only criteria for the residency interview selection.

Try to clear your USMLE Step One on the first attempt. If you have more than one attempt, try to get a better score on USMLE Step 2, at least 220 or above, a 3-digit score. However, if you have a moderate score on step two, try to complete your USMLE step three before submitting the rank order list so that the program will know you have already completed all USMLE exams.

Do I need a USMLE step 3 score to apply?

You do not need a step 3 score to apply for residency. Before the end of residency graduation, you should be able to complete your step three. However, if you have an attempt on step one and/or step two, then the program has no idea whether you will be able to complete your step three or not. So that goes in a negative direction. In that situation, it is advisable to complete the step 3 exam if possible.

To summarize, try to have a first attempt pass on USMLE Step 1 and a decent score on Step 2. But if you have a moderate score on step 2, try to have a step three score.

Vis Tip: USMLE Step 3 is not a criterion for application or for the selection process, but it will boost your application. It carries more weight once you have completed all three USMLE exams.

4. **Letters of recommendation:**

Having at least two specialty-specific letters from attending physicians who have academic appointments or from a program director carries tremendous weight in receiving an interview call.

However, if you don't have a specialty-specific letter, at least try to have some other specialty letters from US-based physicians. For international medical graduates who don't do any clinical rotations in the US, it's challenging to find rotations to get letters of recommendation from US physicians. If you're unable to get a US physician letter of recommendation, at least upload letters from your home country or from your home medical school.

Vis Tip: The weightage of your application will differ based on what you are submitting.

5. **Academic/Research performance:**

Having academic interests like publications and book chapters is also important.

6. **Deans Letter or MSPE (Medical Student Performance Evaluation):**

MSPE carries some weight because it summarizes all your activities during the medical school academic and non-academic. Your dean is highly recommending you for any program, but the downside is that the program will only see your medical school transcript first. They can only download your Deans Letter or MSPE after November, so they must wait until November.

Personal statement:

It is important to know what to include and what not to include in your personal statement. Having a more personalized story carries more weight.

How has your medical school experience shaped you?

What factors contributed to selecting a specialty?

What are you going to bring to the program?

What are you going to contribute to the specialty?

Vis Tip: Having a clear idea, clearer path, and clear vision will place you in a higher position to land you a good interview in a good program.

c. What are the top 3 criteria to get an interview?

The top three I want to recommend are:

- Your USMLE performance

- Your clerkship performance

- Your personalized letters of recommendation

d. Waiving right to see letter of recommendation:

If you waive your right to see a particular letter from an attending physician, that letter carries significant weight because the programs think that those are authentic letters coming directly from the program directors or attending physicians, so that carries a tremendous weight.

e. Do USMLE scores and the number of interviews matter?

You need to understand that having 1-2 interviews doesn't mean that you have no chance of getting into any residency training, and at the same time, having 20 or 30 interviews doesn't mean that your resident spot is already reserved.

The same thing goes with the USMLE scores. If your USMLE scores are low or modest, or if you have more attempts on the USMLE, it doesn't mean that you have no chance of getting into a residency program.

At the same time, if you have high 99s or high three-digit scores like 260 on the USMLE, it doesn't mean that your residency spot is already reserved for you. Please don't be under that impression. You must understand that instead of competing with thousands of applicants, now you're only competing with maybe less than 100 applicants in that residency program once you receive the interview call, so that's the good news. Congratulations. You have already achieved the most important step in this residency application process.

Vis Tip: All you need is one interview to get into a program!

Conclusion:

Every program interview selection criterion is different. The way each factor carries weight for that program is also different. Please consider this as general advice.

Key points:

- *Maintain patience after submitting an application.*
- *Submit a complete application with all necessary documents.*
- *Review program selection criteria before application.*
- *Having all 3 USMLE scores will boost your application.*
- *US letters of recommendation carry more weight.*
- *Hands-on clinical experience is given higher priority in the selection process.*
- *High USMLE scores carry the greatest advantage.*

Chapter 6: Interview preparation and interview

Once you have submitted your ERAS application, you must check your ERAS inbox often for any communication messages from the programs.

a. **Scheduling interview:**

As soon as you receive an email or a message from a program saying that they are interested in scheduling an interview with you, jump right on, grab your phone, and call the program to schedule that interview soon because the programs do not want to wait too long. If you tell the program you're going to get back to the program or you need some more time to decide the interview date, then they might move on and give that option to someone else. You don't want to miss that opportunity. So, go ahead and schedule that interview and lock the interview date first. If you have any conflict in the future, then you can call the program to reschedule or even cancel it. But you need to jump right on and lock that interview day. That's the first thing you need to do.

Vis Tip: Do not delay or postpone scheduling an interview.

b. **Program signaling:**

By this time the programs already have some idea about who you are, where you are coming from, and what your interests are. What are you bringing to the residency program?

ERAS has introduced a new feature called Program Signaling. It means that you can tell the program that, hey, I'm interested in doing my residency in your program. I'm not just coming for the interview, but I'm genuinely interested in your program. The program will have some idea about those candidates who are genuinely interested in their program. Depending on your specialty, you have different program signaling options. Please check with ERAS to see how many programs you can signal. Program signaling will give the program some idea about your genuine interest in the program.

List of programs participating in program signaling and their allotted slots:

- Anesthesiology (5 gold, 10 silver signals)
- Child Neurology & Neurodevelopmental Disabilities (3 signals)
- Dermatology (3 gold, 25 silver signals)
- Diagnostic Radiology & Interventional Radiology (6 gold, 6 silver signals)
- Emergency Medicine (5 signals)
- Family Medicine (5 signals)
- General Surgery (15 signals)
- Internal Medicine (3 gold, 12 silver signals)
- Internal Medicine and Psychiatry (2 signals)
- Neurological Surgery (25 signals)
- Neurology (8 signals)
- Orthopedic Surgery (30 signals)
- Otolaryngology (25 signals)
- Pathology (5 signals)
- Pediatrics (5 signals)
- Physical Medicine and Rehabilitation (8 signals)
- Public Health and General Preventive Medicine (3 signals)
- Psychiatry (10 signals)
- Radiation Oncology (4 signals)
- Thoracic Surgery (3 signals)
- Transitional Year (12 signals)

c. **Preparation is the key:**

You need to do your own homework and research about the program and the department that you are going for an interview.

Know about the program/hospital:

- Who is the chairman?
- who is the program director?
- who are the attending physicians?
- Who are the chief residents?
- Are there any special clinical programs in the department?
- Any research projects going on in the department?
- You need to have a clear idea about the program. Please just don't blindly go and attend the interview.

d. **Know your application:**

You should thoroughly prepare for all the important topics that you have mentioned in your CV or in your ERAS application. Any programs or any research projects that you're working on, clinical experiences, challenging cases, and so on. When they ask you some questions during the interview, you should be able to clearly talk about those points without hesitation.

Vis Tip: It is important that you go to the interview fully prepared

e. **Virtual vs. in-person interview:**

Virtual interview:

After the pandemic, most of the interviews have turned into virtual ones. However, there are some interviews that are conducted in person.

Be prepared for the virtual interview day:

- Make sure you have a good working laptop.
- Good power cable
- Good Internet connection

- Make sure that your family knows that you have an important day in your life.
- Have a secluded place for yourself to complete the interview process successfully.
- Keep away all the electronic devices in switch-off mode.
- If you have children or pets, make sure you have arrangements to take care of them for you.
- Make sure you have professional attire and that you are well-groomed and sharp-looking.
- Print out your ERAS application, CV, and any other research articles or papers that you want to discuss.
- Make sure you have a list of questions that you want to ask the interviewers about the program or about the residency training.
- Have a printed copy of the interview day agenda in front of you.
- Have a notepad, a couple of pens, and a water bottle.

In-person interview:
- Make sure that your family knows that you have an important day in your life.
- Keep away all the electronic devices in switch-off mode.
- If you have children or pets, make sure you have arrangements to take care of them for you.
- Make sure you have professional attire and that you are well-groomed and sharp-looking.
- Print out your ERAS application, CV, and any other research articles or papers that you want to discuss.
- Make sure you have a list of questions that you want to ask the interviewers about the program or about the residency training.
- Have a printed copy of the interview day agenda.

- Have an office file, a notepad, a couple of pens, and a water bottle.

f. Know the pre-interview day agenda:

Are they planning for a pre-interview dinner with the residents?

What time you should attend and where you should go for the pre-interview dinner?

What is the dress code for the dinner?

Who will be attending the dinner, and what are their names?

You do not want to miss a pre-interview dinner with the residents.

g. Know about your interview day:

The most important thing is that you should know about the interview agenda and what your interview day looks like.

1. **Interview day:**
- You do not want to go late to the morning report, or you do not want to miss the presentation by the program director. It doesn't look good on you.
- Make sure you reach the city where the interview takes place the day before, not on the day of the interview, so that you get some good rest.
- Familiarize yourself with the place and know how to reach the place where the interview takes place.
- Prepare important documents you must carry. Make sure that you carry any research projects. Anything that you want to show the program director to improve your chances of getting into the program. Those are the things you usually carry with you on the day of the interview.

- Make sure that you have professional attire, nicely pressed. Look professional and sharp.
- Make sure you reach there at least 15 minutes before so that you're not trying to find the interview place at the last minute.

2. **General interview day agenda:**

- It starts with a morning breakfast presentation from the program director.
- After the presentation, they might invite you to go to the morning report to interact with the residents and to experience the didactics.
- After that, there will be interviews, usually between the program director, the chairman, at least two attending physicians or one attending physician, and one chief resident.
- There will be four or five people who will be interviewing you on that day.
- Every interview is important because each person will give a score on a scoring sheet. All the scoring sheets are presented to the program director at the end of the interview day.
- Please make sure that you treat all the individual interviews as an important component for a well-rounded and successful interview day.

3. **Embrace 4 important qualities or 4Es:**

- Be eager
- Be enthusiastic
- Be excited and
- Be empathetic.

4. **Reject or refuse four Ds:**

- Don't look disappointed
- Don't be discouraged
- Don't be distracted
- Don't be dejected.

5. **Things to remember:**

- Even though there might be gaps in your CV or on your application, you're not going to worry about those things at that moment.
- You must live in the moment.
- You must leave a good impression, that's the goal for the interview day.
- Forget about the outcome of the interview, you must give your best performance in the interview.

h. What to expect from the interviewers?

The interviewers are not going to ask you too many questions about your attempts on your exams or any gaps in your CV.

They're not going to ask you about glucose metabolism, sodium-potassium channels, cardiac physiology, or brain localization.

What are they looking for in a candidate?

- Attitude
- Dedication
- Hardworking nature
- Time management
- Conflict resolution
- Being able to work in a team

- Being able to get things done
- Being able to uplift other people
- Effective communication with the patient and family members
- Being empathetic.
- They might ask you some questions about an interesting case or an interesting situation and how you handled it.
- What are your strengths and weaknesses?
- How can you overcome the stress?
- How can you manage the stress or long hours?

i. Your interview goal:

At the end of the interview day, you should leave an everlasting impression on the program and on the program director. Even after you leave that place after the interview, they should keep thinking about you. They should think that this is the candidate I want in my program. That's the kind of impression that you should leave on the program.

j. Taking notes:

As soon as you reach your hotel room or airport, make sure you take note of all the important things that happened on the interview day, the people you met, their names, and all the things that you learned—all the positives and negatives about the program.

When you're preparing your rank order list, interview notes will guide you in making appropriate decisions regarding where to rank each program.

k. Thank you note:

Once you go home in the next 2-3 days, you might want to send a thank you letter to the program director and all the interviewers saying that you really enjoyed the interview and learned about the program. Please write personalized letters. Please do not copy and paste standard letter templates. It doesn't look good. That's why it's important to take notes after the interview. This information will help you to write a personalized letter. Do not forget to thank the program coordinators because they work hard in the background to get your application to the reviewers, schedule interviews, and print all your documents.

To whom should you send thank you letters?

Program director, chairman, attendings, chief residents, and program coordinator so that you're in the good books.

Key points:

- *Be eager and enthusiastic, don't look disappointed.*
- *Dress appropriately and look sharp.*
- *Know about the program and program agenda*
- *Be on time and be courteous with all the staff*
- *Leave an ever-lasting impression on the program*
- *Take good notes right after the interview ends*
- *Send personalized thank you notes to all the interviewers and program coordinators.*

Chapter 7: Rank order list

a. At the end of each interview, you must take notes.

- What is your experience with the interview?
- What are the positives about the program?
- What are the negatives about the program?

Keep notes after every program interview so that you have notes for all the interviews and all the programs at the end of the interview season.

b. Thank you note: Rank order list

When you're sending a thank you letter to the program director, you can mention in that letter that you're ranking the program high on the rank order list. At the same time, the program director can also send you an email saying that they liked you during the interview. The program director might say that the program wants to rank you high on their rank order list. I advise you not to take these words too seriously, as they may not be legally binding if not documented in a contract or agreement. Before submitting the final rank order list, the program can change its mind. They may not rank you high, or you can change your mind. You may not rank the program high, so don't take these words too seriously.

We will discuss an example. Let's assume that you applied to Physical Medicine & Rehabilitation as your primary specialty. You received ten interviews. Out of 10 interviews, three interviews are for a categorical program that offers four-year training in your specialty. However, seven of the interviews are for advanced Physical Medicine & Rehabilitation residencies that only offer second, third, and 4th-year residency training. In this situation, you need a first-year residency (internship) training before starting advanced training (PGY2).

Let's assume, for that first-year internship, you applied for one-year training programs. Let's say you received ten internship interviews. These internship interviews might be for a transitional one-year program, a preliminary surgery one-year program, or a preliminary internal medicine one-year program. With that, you have ten physical medicine and rehab interviews and ten internship interviews. In total, you have 20 interviews for this season.

Once you have completed all the interviews, you need to go through the notes for every program and the interview experience.

c. How to rank the programs: GF Index/score

I came up with the concept of the GF Index or GF score. Here is a sample GF scorecard:

Program	Interview experience (max 5 pts)	What do you think about the program (max 5 pts)	What program thinks about you (max 5 pts)	Based on your application what is your chance of matching (max 5 pts)	Total GUT FEELING SCORE GF score (max 20 pts)

For each specialty, in this example, the Physical Medicine and Rehabilitation residency program, create a table like the above, and you add all the ten programs from top to bottom. Create another list for internship programs. On the first sheet for the Physical Medicine and Rehabilitation, for each program, grade them under four categories. The first category is: How was your interview experience? Give a maximum of five points. The second category—what do you personally think about the program? Is this the program you want to do your residency in for the next four years or three years? Give a maximum of five points.

The third category is: What does the program think about you? Give a maximum of five points. The 4th category is based on your application: Do you think that you have a high chance of matching into this program? Give a maximum of five points. When you combine all this together, you will get your final score, which I call a GF score. This is your gut feeling score with a maximum of 20 points. If there is a conflict or tie between two programs, program A gets 20 points. Program B got 20 points, then review the notes for those two programs and then take a real close look to see what are the most important things that you like in each of those programs and then try to place higher or lower. Once you have the GF scores in the final column, then change the order of the programs in the list.

Repeat the same process for internship programs too. In this way, you're not randomly assigning the rankings on the rank order list. Once you have done this homework, you will have two lists, one for your primary specialty and one for your internship. But if you're applying to two different specialties, you may need to have two separate lists.

d. NRMP account:

Create an account on the National Residency Matching Program (NRMP) website. Remember that the ERAS application or ERAS account does not give you automatic access to the NRMP account. You need to create a new account using your USMLE ID on the NRMP website (National Residency Match Program). Once you create that account, you will get access to their R three system (Registration, Ranking, and Result system).

e. Other MATCH agencies:

In addition to NRMP, there are other match agencies for certain specialties. Please refer to Appendix A.

Match programs

National Residency Matching Program – www.nrmp.org

SF Match (for certain specialties including ophthalmology, plastic surgery, and other fellowships) – www.sfmatch.org

Urology Match – www.auanet.org

f. Rank order lists:

Create your primary rank order list for your primary specialty, in this example, Physical Medicine & Rehabilitation. Enter all the programs in the order that you want based on the GF scorecard. Now create a supplemental rank order list for your internship programs. Enter all the programs in the order based on the GF scorecard. Both lists must be separate. You can either save them or you can sign those lists. Remember that if you don't cross the due date set for submitting the list, you can edit the lists even after signing your rank list. You can add programs or delete programs. You can change the order as many times as you want until the deadline. But once you cross the due date for submitting the rank order list, you can no longer make changes from the NRMP website account.

If you think that you desperately need to make changes after the deadline but before the match day, then you must personally call the NRMP National Residency Match Program and discuss with them to see how they can help you make those changes before the actual match day.

That's how you make an educated decision based on your performance, based on what you think about the program, and rank your programs appropriately.

g. For couples:

If you are a couple and you wish to stay in the same program or within a similar geographical area, you should choose the couples match option when you're uploading the rank order list

h. Primary Vs. Supplemental rank order list:

You must know the difference between a primary rank order list and a supplemental rank order list. On the primary rank order list, you can include any type of program. It might be a categorical program, a preliminary program, an advanced program, or a program related to different specialties.

However, if you have uploaded an advanced PGY 2 program on the primary rank order list, then you should have a supplemental rank order list with a corresponding preliminary program. Then only will you be able to match into both advanced and preliminary programs during the same match.

i. NRMP registration deadline:

The deadline is March 5th (dates might vary each year). That's the last day that you can enroll for the match process. That's also the last day that you can upload and make any changes to your rank order list. After March 5th you will no longer be able to upload any rank order list or even enroll for the match program for the current year.

j. Programs not to include on final rank order list:

If you have interviewed at a certain program and for some reason you don't like that program, you don't want to be doing residency in that program. Please do not include that program in your final rank order list.

What happens is when you include a program in the final rank order list for the match and you sign the rank order list. That means you are getting into a binding agreement with the NRMP match process rules and regulations. If at all you match into that program, then you agree to accept the offer from the program. That's why if you do not like certain programs that you interviewed, please do not include them in your final rank order list.

k. Maximizing your chances of a match:

If you have no reservations about any program that you interviewed with and your goal for this match year is to match into any program, then to maximize your chances of matching into any program, you should include every program that you have interviewed with. In that way, you are maximizing your chances of residency.

Vis tip: *Rank all the programs that you attended an interview to maximize the chance of a match.*

l. What to include on the primary rank order list:

I recommend that you include all your transitional programs, preliminary programs, categorical programs, and advanced programs (even from different specialties) on your primary rank order list to maximize your chances of matching into a program.

m. More resources and information:

I want you all to make sure that you have enrolled on the NRMP website. There are plenty of resources on the nrmp.org website. I want all the residency applicants to be familiar with these resources on the website.

Key points:

- *Include all programs on the primary rank order list*
- *Use the GF score card to rank programs based on your interview performance and program performance.*
- *Create a supplemental list if you are ranking advanced programs on primary rank order list*
- *Do not include any program that you do not like*
- *Choose a couple's match if you and your partner want to stay close.*
- *Follow the timelines, NRMP account registration is needed to participate in the match.*

Chapter 8: NRMP MATCH

a. **NRMP match algorithm:**

Let's take an example so it's easier to understand how the NRMP match algorithm works. Program A interviewed 100 candidates for the current year, and the residency committee has decided to rank the top 15 candidates for their five spots. You can ask me why they are ranking 15 candidates when they only have five spots. The reason is not every candidate wants to accept the offer from that program A. To maximize their chances of matching candidates into their open spots, programs usually rank more candidates. Program A decided to rank 15 candidates for five spots. That means they're ranking three candidates for each spot.

1. **NRMP match algorithm for the candidates:**

Dr. Will submitted the rank order list. The number one choice for Dr. Will is Program A, and the number two choice is Program B. Once Dr. Will submits the rank order list, the NRMP match algorithm works in such a way that it will always try to match the candidate to their number one choice program. For Dr. Will, the number one choice program is program A. The NRMP match algorithm will try to match Dr. Will to program A.

You must keep in mind that program A also should rank Dr. Will high. Then only the match happens. But remember, there were several other candidates who also interviewed for the program A. They also ranked that program high. Because that program did not rank Dr. Will high, the match did not happen between Dr. Will and program A.

What the algorithm does is, now it pushes that program A all the way down on Dr. Will's rank order list. His second choice is program B. Now program B has become his top choice. The matching algorithm will try to match Dr. Will with Program B. It keeps going through the entire list of programs on the primary rank order list submitted by Dr. Will until it finds a match for him. That's how the rank algorithm works for the candidate.

2. NRMP match algorithm for the programs:

If you look at the program side, in this example, program A. The top choice on their 15 top candidates rank order list is, let's assume, Dr. Y. However, Dr. Y decided to go to some other program other than Program A. That means for program A, Doctor Y is no longer their top choice because Dr. Y already accepted a position at some other place.

Now the second candidate on the program's list becomes their top choice. That's how the NRMP match algorithm works for the residency programs.

b. NRMP match:

On March 17th (dates might vary each year) of the current ERAS cycle, the candidates will receive an email with the match result - matched, partially matched, or did not match. These are the three outcomes of the main match.

c. Outcomes of the primary NRMP match:
- Matched completely
- Did not match
- Partially matched

Partially matched means the candidate might have applied to an advanced position and a preliminary position. However, the candidate has been matched into an advanced program but not into a preliminary program.

If you are matched into a categorical program or a preliminary program on your primary rank order list, the matching algorithm stops there. However, if you matched into an advanced program on your primary rank order list, then the matching algorithm will run your supplementary rank order list and will try to match you for the PGY1 or a preliminary position. In that way, you will have both a PGY2 or advanced position and a PGY1 or a preliminary position.

Keep in mind that if you're applying for a PGY2 or an advanced position, that means that you are starting that PGY2 on July 1st of the following year, not the current match year. You need a PGY1 or preliminary position starting on July 1st of the current match year so that you can complete the PGY1 year and then move on to the PGY2 year.

Please note that both the programs and the candidates must submit their final rank order list. Please be advised that the programs may not submit all the candidates that they interviewed on the final rank order list. The programs might select only top candidates depending on the number of residency positions available in the program.

d. Match Day:

March 21st (dates might vary every year) is the MATCH Day. On that day, you will receive an email notifying you which program and what specialty you matched into. All the medical schools will also celebrate their medical school students with offer letters.

Key points:

- Both the candidate and the program must submit the final rank order list before the due date.
- The candidate must submit a primary as well as a supplemental rank order list if applying for an advanced position.
- Programs may not include all the candidates they interviewed on the final rank order list, only top candidates.

Chapter 9: Supplemental MATCH and off cycle positions

On the evening of March 17th (dates might vary every year), NRMP will post all the unfilled positions. You can access those positions from your NRMP, R three system. On March 18th, you will have the option to apply to these unfilled positions if you're partially matched or if you're not matched at all.

a. S.O.A.P (Supplemental Offer and Application Program):

SOAP is your last chance to get into a residency position for that ERAS season. You can apply to a maximum of 30 unfilled positions using your ERAS account. On March 19th, the programs will review applications for the unfilled positions. On March 20th programs start sending offer letters via ERAS inbox for unfilled positions. You can either accept the offer or you can wait for the next round of offers. There will be four rounds in which all the offers will be made for the unfilled positions on March 20th. By the evening of March 20th, all the residency programs will try to fill all the unfilled positions.

b. Main match Vs. supplemental match:

You should know the difference between the main match and a supplemental match, also called S.O.A.P. The main match is something for which you submit your rank order list by March 5th of that cycle. Once the programs and the residency candidates submit the rank order list, the main match will happen right after the final match deadline, which is March 5th (dates might vary each cycle).

After the final match, you will have an option to apply for a supplemental match, also called S.O.A.P. (Supplemental Offer and Application Program), for unfilled positions if you are not matched or if you are partially matched during the main match.

Once both the main match and supplemental match are completed, then only the match day happens, which is March 21st (dates might vary each cycle) for that match season. On that day you will know exactly what specialty and where you matched.

Vis Tip*: If you did not match or only partially matched in the main match, then do not hesitate to apply for the supplemental match.*

c. Off-cycle positions or non-ERAS positions:

Residency programs might not fill all their positions by the end of the main match and the supplemental match. Even after the supplemental match offers, there might be some positions that are vacant.

You must contact the programs directly to see if there are any open spots available outside the ERAS season that they're trying to fill before June. Because all the residency programs start on July 1st. There might be some off-cycle programs that might start later in the year. You might have to check directly with the programs to see if they still have any sports available after the March deadline for the match.

Vis Tip: *If you did not find a position even in a supplemental match, keep contacting programs for any unfilled positions for that year.*

How to apply to off cycle positions:

Once you confirm that a program has a vacancy outside the ERAS season, you can send in the paper documents and then submit your application outside the ERAS application before the start date for that year. The interview will take place depending on when the program wants that candidate to start.

Please refer to Appendix A.

Non-ERAS /Non ACGME positions:

AMA - https://www.ama-assn.org/medical-students/preparing-residency/non-acgme-open-residency-fellowship-positions

Off-cycle residency positions:

Vacant, unfilled, new, and other types of open positions throughout the year

www.residentswap.org

AMA FindAResident for year-round open residency and fellowship positions –

https://students-residents.aamc.org/findaresident/findaresident-search-tool

Key dates: *(Dates might vary each year)*

- *March 5th: Final day to register for NRMP match account*
- *March 5th: Final day for the candidates to submit the final rank order list.*
- *March 17th: matched, partially matched, unmatched results sent to the candidates*
- *March 17th: unfilled positions list posted*
- *March 18th: SOAP or supplemental match application opens*
- *March 19th: Programs start reviewing applications for unfilled positions*
- *March 20th: Supplemental match offers sent to candidates in 4 cycles throughout the day.*
- *March 20th: SOAP ends by that evening*
- *March 21st: Match Day. Candidates receive emails regarding the program and specialty matched.*

Chapter 10: Visa Requirements for IMGs

a. B-1/ B-2 or a visitor visa:

If you are an international medical graduate (IMG) also termed a foreign medical graduate (FMG) residing outside the United States, you might have to come to the US mainly for three reasons.

- Clerkship program or an externship program.
- USMLE step 3 exam before residency training.
- In person residency interview.

After the pandemic, the USMLE program requirements have changed. There is no longer a step 2 CS. USMLE step 3 is the only exam for which you might have to come to the United States if you're planning to take that exam before starting your residency training.

Most of the programs are doing only virtual interviews after the pandemic. There are only a few programs that are asking candidates to attend in-person interviews. If any program requires you to come to the United States for an in-person interview, then you might have to apply for a visa.

In these three situations: an externship or a clerkship, a USMLE step 3 exam before residency training, and an in-person residency interview, you must apply for a B-1/ B-2 or a visitor visa.

b. Visa waiver program:

There are certain countries that come under a Visa Waiver Program. If your home country comes under a Visa Waiver Program, you do not have to apply for a visa. All you need is a valid passport and a letter either from that program where you're going for a clerkship or an interview or a letter from ECFMG for the USMLE exam. At the port of entry into the United States, the visa officer will review those documents and grant up to 90 days or three months.

If you do not qualify for a Visa Waiver Program, then you need to apply to the US Consulate in your country for a B-/B-2 visa. Please check with your US consulate regarding the wait times for an interview and visa stamping because the process might be delayed. You want to make sure you get those documents on time.

c. Once you have matched into a residency position:

There are mainly two pathways that you can take to start your residency training in the United States. The first pathway is the J-1 visa program, which is the Exchange Visitor Visa Program, and the second pathway is the H-1B visa program.

1. Requirements for the J-1 Visa program:

Completion of USMLE step one, step two.

ECFMG certificate

A letter from the program that you have matched into residency.

The J-1 visa is sponsored by the Education Commission for Foreign Medical Graduates (ECFMG). Most of the residency programs are now preferring or turning to J-1 visa programs because it's much easier for the program, and there's less documentation from the program side. It's all processed by ECFMG. Once you have all the required documents, the ECFMG will issue a certificate that you're eligible to apply for a J-1 visa. They will also issue a Form DS 2019. You need to apply for a statement of need from your home country. The ECFMG will send your visa application packet to the US consulate in your country. Then you must apply for a visa interview and get the visa stamping.

Once you get the J-1 visa, it is usually valid for up to seven years, which is good if you're planning to do fellowship training after residency; you still have the validity on the J-1 visa.

2. Requirements for H1B visa program:

USMLE step one, step two, and step three.

Qualify for any state license requirements.

An acceptance letter from the residency program that you matched into.

In this situation, you might have to come to the United States before starting your residency training on some B1/B2 visa or a visa waiver program to take your USMLE step three exam.

For H-1B aspiring candidates, the residency program that you matched into must process your H-1B application.

With all the required documentation, the program needs to get a labor clearance first and then file your documentation with the USCIS. Then the entire file will be sent to the US consulate in your country. Only then can you apply for a US visa interview and get your H-1B visa stamped. Once your H-1B is approved, it's usually valid for up to six years.

Dependent visa:

If you are coming to the US on a J-1 visa, you can apply for a J-2 (dependent) visa for your spouse and children. Similarly, if you're coming on an H-1B visa, you can apply for an H-4 (dependent) visa for your spouse and children to come along with you.

d. Home country rule:

J-1 visa holders come under an exchange visitor program. Home country rule applies after residency training. That means you must return to your home country for two years after completion of residency training and then apply for a work visa from your home country.

e. J1 visa waiver program:

If you wish to stay in the US on a J1 visa after completion of your residency training, you must do a visa waiver program for at least three years in the United States in a rural area setting before you can convert your J-1 into H-1B work visa.

f. H-1B visa after residency training:

Once you finish your residency training on an H1B visa, you must look for another employer that comes under the H1B visa cap exemption because non-cap-exempt H-1B visas are limited and difficult to get. You must find an employer that comes under the H-1B cap-exempt to convert your H-1B from residency training to your first job right after residency training. Please check wait times or grace periods if you are applying to non-cap exempt jobs after residency training. Working with an experienced immigration attorney is recommended in this situation.

Vis Tip: J1 is easier to get, however, need to fulfill a 3-year visa waiver; opt for H1B if you have an option from your program.

g. Conversion from other visa types within the US:

If you are an IMG already in the United States on an F1 (student visa), you can convert to a J1 or H1B visa for residency training.

If you are an IMG already in the United States on a J1 research visa, you might be able to convert to a J1 residency training visa. Please contact ECFMG for further assistance.

If you are an IMG already in the United States on an H1B visa, you might be able to transfer your H1B to your residency program.

Please contact your residency program or contact an immigration attorney for further assistance.

Please refer to Appendix A.

For International Medical Graduates (IMGs/FMGs):

Educational Commission for Foreign Medical Graduates –

www.ecfmg.org

ECFMG OASIS (Online Applicant Status and Information System) – https://oasis2.ecfmg.org

U.S. Citizenship and Immigration Services: www.uscis.org

J-1 Exchange Visitor Visa Program –

https://j1visa.state.gov/basics/

Key points:

- *A J1 visa is valid for up to 7 years and does not require a step 3 score to apply.*
- *An H1B visa is valid up to 6 years and requires step 3 score to apply.*
- *J1 is an exchange visitor visa - visa waiver or home country rule applies after residency training.*
- *It is possible to convert from F1, J1 research or H1B visa once you match into a residency program.*

Chapter 11: Not matched, now what?

USMLE exams, residency applications, interviews, rank order lists, and the NRMP match—all these steps involve a lot of dedication, hard work, persistence, and, above all, patience. I did not match into my specialty on the first attempt. I never lost hope or confidence. I kept working on bettering myself, improving my CV, and expanding my overall knowledge and outlook on the field. My advice to those who did not match is not to lose hope. Critically review your application and areas where you need to improve while waiting to apply for the next application season. Attend conferences and network with people in the field. Presenting abstracts or posters at conferences is a great way to gain recognition and network with people who want to give you an interview. Keeping yourself up to date with the field and actively working in the areas related to the specialty that you want to go into would greatly improve your chances of matching. If you are not sure about the direction you are heading, then finding a mentor who can help you navigate the path might be a good option.

For IMGs who did not match on 2-3 attempts and are not sure how to proceed, I would like to offer some advice. If you wish to stay in the United States, you need to have some visa status. Finding a master's or PhD program might be a good option that can sponsor an F1 or J1 visa according to the program. You could also apply to postdoctoral positions or paid research positions. Please note that these paid positions are highly competitive. You must go to several university websites to find jobs and apply directly on their websites. You could also find a voluntary research position in any department or in a wet or dry research lab (need some visa status) and work your way up. Please note that voluntary positions do not offer visas; However, some unpaid research positions might offer J-1 research visas. Please make sure to check work restrictions while on visa status. You could also apply to industry-related jobs like medical monitors or clinical liaison jobs at pharmaceutical companies. These are some of the options for IMGs who wish to stay in the United States while pursuing residency options.

Vis Tip: If you are coming to the US on a B1/B2 visa during the interview season, try to schedule all your interviews during that visa period. Also, try to do some observership or gain some experience while you are here before you are required to leave the country.

All these pathways also apply to US medical graduates who did not match or who are looking for some kind of work experience while waiting to apply for the next cycle.

I hope to see you all match into your top choice program and come out with flying colors. All the best.

Key points:

- *Keep yourself up to date and working in the area related to the specialty of your choice.*
- *Keep working on improving your CV.*
- *Critically review your application and areas that need improvement.*
- *Find a mentor that can guide you.*

Chapter 12: Final remarks

I trust that you have acquired valuable information and valuable advice regarding the application process for residency programs and the process of participating in an interview or NRMP match. Please do not hesitate to contact me at **viswanath.aluru@gmail.com** if you have any additional inquiries. I would be delighted to provide you with personal responses to your inquiries or to publish an additional video online that addresses frequently asked questions.

"I hope that all of you have a successful residency"

APPENDIX A

PHYSICIAN RESOURCES AND WEBSITES

APPENDIX A

PHYSCIAN RESOURCES AND WEBSITES

USMLE preparation:

U.S. Medical Licensing examination – www.usmle.org
National Board of Medical Examiner – www.nbme.org
Federation of State Medical Boards – www.fsmb.org
Education Commission for Foreign Medical Graduates – www.ecfmg.org
Kaplan Medical Test Prep – www.kaptest.com
USMLE World – www.uworld.com

ERAS services:
Association of American Medical Colleges – www.aamc.org
Electronic Residency Application Service (ERAS) – www.myeras.aamc.org

Residency program search:
American Medical Association – www.ama.org
AMA FREIDA program directory - https://freida.ama-assn.org
FindAResident search tool - https://systems.aamc.org/findaresident/

Match programs
National Residency Matching Program – www.nrmp.org
SF Match (for certain specialties including Ophthalmology, Plastic Surgery and other fellowships) – www.sfmatch.org
Urology Match – www.auanet.org

Post-Match services:
Supplemental Offer and Match Program (SOAP) –
https://www.nrmp.org/residency-applicants/soap/

Non-ERAS /Non ACGME positions:
AMA - https://www.ama-assn.org/medical-students/preparing-residency/non-acgme-open-residency-fellowship-positions

Off-cycle residency positions:
Vacant, unfilled, new and other types of open positions throughout the year
www.residentswap.org

For International Medical Graduates (IMGs/FMGs):
Educational Commission for Foreign Medical Graduates – www.ecfmg.org
ECFMG OASIS (Online Applicant Status and Information System) –

https://oasis2.ecfmg.org
U.S. Citizenship and Immigration Services: www.uscis.org
J-1 Exchange Visitor Visa Program - https://j1visa.state.gov/basics/

APPENDIX B

ERAS APPLICATION TEMPLATE
ERAS APPLICATION CHECKLIST

APPENDIX B

ERAS Application Template

Please visit aamc.org for more information on the ERAS tools and work sheets
This work sheet can be downloaded electronically at the link below:
https://students-residents.aamc.org/eras-tools-and-worksheets-residency-applicants/eras-tools-and-worksheets-residency-applicants

This template is provided here only for information and understanding purposes

AAMC Account Information
Basic Information
Previous Last Name
Preferred Name
Preferred Pronoun
Preferred Phone*
Mobile Phone
Alternate Phone
Fax
Pager

Address
Current Mailing Address
Permanent Address

Work Authorization
(Required for U.S. & Canadian addresses.)
Are you currently authorized to work in the United States? * Yes No
What is your current work authorization? *
Will you need visa sponsorship through ECFMG (J-1) or the teaching hospital (H-1B) to complete the entirety of your GME training? *
Yes No
If yes, please select the visa(s) for which you will seek sponsorship. Select all that apply. *
H-1B J-1
If no, please identify which status will serve as your basis for work authorization for the entirety
of your GME training without any need for visa sponsorship. Select all that apply.
Match® Information

Yes No
If yes, NRMP ID:
Couples Match Yes No
If yes, partner's name:
Specialties partner is applying to:
Urology Match®
AUA Member Number:

Identification Numbers
USMLE/ECFMG ID:
NBOME ID:
American Osteopathic Association Member Number:
(Required for D.O. applicants.)

Biographic Information
Self-Identification
How do you self-identify? Please list all that apply.

Language Fluency
Please describe your level of proficiency in all the languages you speak.
Native/Near native
Advanced
Good
Fair
Basic
Do you meet or exceed the Advanced level of proficiency in English? Yes No
If you speak a language other than English, which of the languages do you meet or exceed the good level of proficiency?

Military Information
Are you committed to fulfill a U.S. military active-duty service obligation/deferment? * Yes No
If yes, number of years remaining: Branch:
Do you have any other service obligations (e.g., military reserves, public health/state programs)? * Yes No
If yes, describe:
255-character limit

Geographic Preferences
The division preferences section offers you an opportunity to communicate your preference or lack of preference for geographic divisions. Indicate your preference (or lack of preference) for up to three U.S. Census divisions.

Higher Education
This section allows multiple entries for each undergraduate and graduate school you have attached.
Since most non-U.S. educational systems do not follow the U.S. model, almost all students and graduates of international medical schools will indicate "None."
Location*
Field(s) of Study*
Month Year
Institution*
Education Type*
Degree Expected or Earned*
If Yes: Degree
Dates of Attendance: From Month* From Year* To Month* To Year*

Education
Medical Education
This section allows entries for each medical school you have attended.
Country*
Institution*
Degree*
Degree Month*
Degree Year*
Dates of Education
From Month* From Year* To Month* To Year*

Postgraduate Training
Please add an entry for each of your current or prior trainings.
Extensions & Interruptions
Have you had any unplanned professionalism or academic issues in your medical education or training that caused an interruption or extension?

Honors & Awards
Honor Societies
Sigma Phi Status:

Alpha Omega Alpha Status:
Gold Humanism Honor Society Status:

Other Honors or Awards:
Honor or Award Type:
Name:
Description:
Date Received:

Professional Memberships

Selected Experiences
Please identify and describe up to 10 experiences that communicate who you are, what you are passionate about, and what is most important to you.

Organization*
Experience Type*
Position Title*
I am currently working in this role
Start Date* End Date*
Country*
City*
Participation Frequency
Primary Focus Area
Context, Roles, and Responsibilities:
750-character limit
State/Province*
Postal Code*
Setting
Key Characteristics

Selected Experiences | What made this experience meaningful?
Identify and describe up to 3 of the 10 experiences that you found the most meaningful.
Reflect on the experience, why it was meaningful, and how it influenced you. Weave in the focus area or key characteristic you tagged. This should not describe what you did in the experience or list a set of skills that you developed or demonstrated during the experience.
Description:
300-character limit

Impactful Experiences

The following examples can help you decide whether you should respond to the section and what kinds of experiences are appropriate to share on the MyERAS application. Please keep in mind that this is not a fully inclusive list:

- Family background (e.g., first generation to graduate college).
- Financial background (e.g., low-income family, worked to support family growing up, work-study program to pay for college).
- Community setting (e.g., food scarcity, poverty or crime rate, lack of access to medical care).
- Educational experiences (e.g., limited educational opportunities, limited access to advisors or mentors).
- Other general life circumstances (e.g., loss of a family member, serving as a caregiver while working or in school).

750-character limit

Hobbies & Interests

Please provide details regarding your hobbies and interests.
300-character limit

Licenses & Certifications

Please add an entry for any of your state medical licenses.

Additional Questions

Are you able to carry out the responsibilities of a resident, intern, or a fellow in the specialties and at the specific training programs to which you are applying, including the functional requirements, cognitive requirements, and interpersonal and communication requirements with or without reasonable accommodations? *

Has your medical license ever been suspended/revoked/voluntarily terminated? *

Have you been named in a malpractice case? *

Is there anything in your history that would limit your ability to be licensed or would limit your ability to receive hospital privileges? (Note: This section is not intended to solicit information about your health, disability, or family status). *

Have you ever been convicted of a misdemeanor in the United States? *

Have you ever been convicted of a felony in the United States? *

Publications
Add an entry for each of your publications.
 Publication Title*
255 Character Max
Author(s)*
URL*
Publication Date*

Peer-Reviewed Journal Articles/Abstracts

Peer-Reviewed Journal Articles/Abstracts (Other Than Published)

Peer-Reviewed Book Chapter

Scientific Monograph

Poster Presentation

Oral Presentation

Peer-Reviewed Online Publication

Non-Peer-Reviewed Online Publication

DEA Registration

Board Certifications
If other, Board Name:
Certification(s):

Other Certifications
Do you have other medical or health care related certifications?
Certification(s):
Date Received:
Valid Until:

Program Signals
Program signals offer applicants the opportunity to express interest in a residency program at the time of application.

Below are the specialties participating in program signals and their allotted signals.

o Anesthesiology (5 gold, 10 silver signals)
o Child Neurology & Neurodevelopmental Disabilities (3 signals)
o Dermatology (3 gold, 25 silver signals)
o Diagnostic Radiology & Interventional Radiology (6 gold, 6 silver signals)
o Emergency Medicine (5 signals)
o Family Medicine (5 signals)
o General Surgery (15 signals)
o Internal Medicine (3 gold, 12 silver signals)
o Internal Medicine and Psychiatry (2 signals)
o Neurological Surgery (25 signals)
o Neurology (8 signals)
o Orthopedic Surgery (30 signals)
o Otolaryngology (25 signals)
o Pathology (5 signals)
o Pediatrics (5 signals)
o Physical Medicine and Rehabilitation (8 signals)
o Public Health and General Preventive Medicine (3 signals)
o Psychiatry (10 signals)
o Radiation Oncology (4 signals)
o Thoracic Surgery (3 signals)
o Transitional Year (12 signals)

Certification

I certify that the information contained within the MyERAS application is complete and accurate to the best of my knowledge.

APPENDIX B

ERAS APPLICATION CHECKLIST

Request ERAS token from dean's office or ECFMG (IMGs)

Create AAMC account, activate MyERAS using ERAS token

Request letters of recommendation from letter writers

Start searching for programs in your desired specialty

MyERAS account document checklist

- Professional photograph
- Personal statement/s
- Letters of recommendation (non-waived)
- Medical Student Performance Evaluation (MSPE)
- ECFMG certificate (IMGs)
- Medical school transcript
- USMLE or COMPLEX transcript

Save programs under MyERAS account and attached appropriate documents

Apply to program when ERAS application opens

Monitor document tracking and ERAS inbox for messages, interview calls

Register with a Match service (NRMP, Urology, SF Match) based on your specialty

Finalize and submit rank order list- primary and supplementary if needed.

Check Match result.

Participate in S.O.A.P if partially matched or unmatched.

APPENDIX C

STATE SPECIFIC REQUIREMENTS FOR INITIAL MEDICAL LICENSURE

APPENDIX C

STATE SPECIFIC REQUIREMENTS FOR INITIAL MEDICAL LICENSURE

FSMB reviews and updates this information annually and/or at the request of a board. We strongly encourage you to use this as a guide and to contact the board for the most recent information.

Following data is provided only for the information and understanding of requirements.

This information is available electronically on the FSMB website at
https://www.fsmb.org/step-3/state-licensure/

Please contact Federation of State Medical Boards for up-to-date information and further queries:
https://www.fsmb.org/contact-a-state-medical-board/

Alabama
Accepts FCVS
Number of attempts at Licensing Exam
4th attempt at USMLE Step 3 following proof of formal training after the 3rd attempt
10 attempts at all USMLE Steps
No limit on COMLEX
Minimum Postgraduate Training Required
1year ACGME training for US grads
2 years ACGME training for IMG's
Time Limit for Completing Licensing Examination Sequence
7 years to successfully complete all USMLE Steps
No limit on COMLEX (if board certified by one of the ABMS approved boards can complete all parts in10 years)

Alaska
Accepts FCVS
Number of attempts at Licensing Exam
2 attempts per USMLE Step
2 attempts per COMLEX Level
Minimum Postgraduate Training Required
2 years

3 years IMG
Time Limit for Completing Licensing Examination Sequence
7 years to complete USMLE
10 years for MD/PhD candidates
7 years to complete COMLEX

Arizona Medical
Accepts FCVS
Number of attempts at Licensing Exam
No limit on USMLE
Minimum Postgraduate Training Required
1 year
3 years IMG
Time Limit for Completing Licensing Examination Sequence
7 years to complete USMLE if initial licensure
No limit if already licensed.

Arizona Osteopathic
Accepts FCVS
Number of attempts at Licensing Exam
Contact the board for information
Minimum Postgraduate Training Required
1 year
Time Limit for Completing Licensing Examination Sequence
Contact the board for information

Arkansas
Accepts FCVS
Number of attempts at Licensing Exam
3 attempts per USMLE Step
3 attempts per COMLEX Level
Minimum Postgraduate Training Required
1 year
3 years IMG unless currently enrolled in training program through University of Arkansas for Medical Sciences.
Time Limit for Completing Licensing Examination Sequence
No limit on USMLE or COMLEX
California Medical
Limited acceptance of FCVS
Number of attempts at Licensing Exam

4 attempts at USMLE Step 3
Minimum Postgraduate Training Required
1 year
2 years IMG
Time Limit for Completing Licensing Examination Sequence
Passing scores on a written/computerized exam shall be valid for a period of 10 years from the month of the examination.

California Osteopathic
Limited Acceptance of FCVS
Number of attempts at Licensing Exam
No limit on COMLEX
Minimum Postgraduate Training Required
1 year
Time Limit for Completing Licensing Examination Sequence
No limit on COMLEX

Colorado
Accepts FCVS
Number of attempts at Licensing Exam
No limit on USMLE
No information available on COMLEX
Minimum Postgraduate Training Required
1 year
Time Limit for Completing Licensing Examination Sequence
7 years from first sitting to complete USMLE or COMLEX
10 years for MD/PhD or DO/PhD candidates

Connecticut
Accepts FCVS
Number of attempts at Licensing Exam
No limit on USMLE
No limit on COMLEX
Minimum Postgraduate Training Required
2 years
Time Limit for Completing Licensing Examination Sequence
No limit on USMLE
No limit on COMLEX

Delaware
Accepts FCVS
Number of attempts at Licensing Exam
No more than 6 attempts to pass each step
Minimum Postgraduate Training Required
1 year
3 years IMG
Time Limit for Completing Licensing Examination Sequence
7 years to complete USMLE

Washington, DC
Accepts FCVS
Number of attempts at Licensing Exam
3 attempts at USMLE Step 3; After which one additional year of postgraduate training is required.
No limit on COMLEX
Minimum Postgraduate Training Required
1 year
3 years IMG
Time Limit for Completing Licensing Examination Sequence
7 years to complete USMLE; No limit on COMLEX

Florida Medical
Highly recommends FCVS
Number of attempts at Licensing Exam
No limit on USMLE
Minimum Postgraduate Training Required
1 year
2 years IMG
Time Limit for Completing Licensing Examination Sequence
No limit on USMLE

Florida Osteopathic
Highly recommends FCVS
Number of attempts at Licensing Exam
Contact the board for information
Minimum Postgraduate Training Required
1 year in an AOA-approved program
Time Limit for Completing Licensing Examination Sequence
No limit on COMLEX

Georgia
Accepts FCVS
Number of attempts at Licensing Exam
3 attempts per USMLE Step
No limit on COMLEX
Minimum Postgraduate Training Required
1 year
1 year if IMG is on list
3 years IMG if not on list
Time Limit for Completing Licensing Examination Sequence
7 years to complete USMLE
9 years to complete USMLE if in MD/PhD program
No limit on COMLEX

Guam
Accepts FCVS
Number of attempts at Licensing Exam
No limit on USMLE or COMPLEX
Minimum Postgraduate Training Required
3 years of progressive postgraduate medical training
Time Limit for Completing Licensing Examination Sequence
No limit on the USMLE or COMLEX

Hawaii
Accepts FCVS
Number of attempts at Licensing Exam
No limit on USMLE or COMLEX
Minimum Postgraduate Training Required
1 year
2 years IMG
Time Limit for Completing Licensing Examination Sequence
No limit on USMLE or COMLEX

Idaho
Accepts FCVS
Requires Uniform Application
Number of attempts at Licensing Exam

Failure to pass USMLE after 2 attempts may lead to Board interview or evaluation
No limit on COMLEX
Minimum Postgraduate Training Required
1 year
3 years IMG (can be licensed after 2 years if in good standing with Idaho residency training program, and has signed an agreement to complete residency in Idaho)
Time Limit for Completing Licensing Examination Sequence
No limit on USMLE or COMLEX

Illinois
Accepts FCVS
Number of attempts at Licensing Exam
5 attempts at all USMLE Steps combined
5 attempts at COMLEX Levels combined
Minimum Postgraduate Training Required
24 months of training
Time Limit for Completing Licensing Examination Sequence
7 years to complete USMLE
No limit on COMLEX

Indiana
Accepts FCVS
Number of attempts at Licensing Exam
3 attempts per USMLE Step
5 attempts per COMLEX Level
Minimum Postgraduate Training Required
1 year
2 years IMG
Time Limit for Completing Licensing Examination Sequence
10 years to complete USMLE
7 years to complete COMLEX

Iowa
Accepts FCVS
check
Utilizes Uniform Application
Number of attempts at Licensing Exam
6 attempts at both USMLE Step 1 and 2

3 attempts at USMLE Step 3
6 attempts at both COMLEX Levels 1 and 2
3 attempts at COMLEX Level 3
3 years of approved postgraduate training required if outside the attempt limit.
Minimum Postgraduate Training Required
1 year
2 years IMG
Time Limit for Completing Licensing Examination Sequence
10 years to complete USMLE or COMLEX
10 years for MD/PhD or DO/PhD candidates. Note: Board certification by ABMS or AOA is required if the applicant has not met the specified time.

Kansas
Accepts FCVS
Number of attempts at Licensing Exam
3+ attempts at USMLE Step 3 or COMLEX Level 3
Minimum Postgraduate Training Required
1 year
3 years IMG (minimum 2 years in an ACGME approved program)
Time Limit for Completing Licensing Examination Sequence
10 years to complete USMLE or COMLEX

Kentucky
Requires FCVS
Number of attempts at Licensing Exam
Step or Level 1-4 attempts
Step or Level 2 CK-4 attempts
Step or Level 2 CS-4 attempts
Step or Level 3-4 attempts
Minimum Postgraduate Training Required
2 years
Time Limit for Completing Licensing Examination Sequence
No limit on USMLE or COMLEX

Louisiana
Requires FCVS
Number of attempts at Licensing Exam
No limit at USMLE Step 1 or COMLEX Level 1
4 attempts each at USMLE Steps 2 and 3 or COMLEX Levels 2 and 3
Minimum Postgraduate Training Required

2 years
Time Limit for Completing Licensing Examination Sequence
10 years to complete USMLE or COMLEX

Maine Medical
Requires FCVS
Number of attempts at Licensing Exam
3 attempts at USMLE Step 3. More than 3 attempts require a request for a waiver.
Minimum Postgraduate Training Required
US/Canadian medical school graduates who graduated after July 1, 2004 must complete 3 years of ACGME accredited postgraduate training. (Those who graduated before July 1, 2004 are only required to complete 2 years of ACGME accredited PGT.) IMGs 3 years of ACGME accredited.
Time Limit for Completing Licensing Examination Sequence
7 years to complete exam sequence (NBME, USMLE, and FLEX) More than 7 years requires a waiver.

Maine Osteopathic
Accepts FCVS
Number of attempts at Licensing Exam
3 attempts at each Step/Level
Minimum Postgraduate Training Required
1 year in AOA approved program
Time Limit for Completing Licensing Examination Sequence
No limit on COMLEX

Maryland
Requires FCVS
Number of attempts at Licensing Exam
Unlimited attempts at each USMLE Step or COMLEX Level
Minimum Postgraduate Training Required
1 year
2 years IMG
Time Limit for Completing Licensing Examination Sequence
No time limit. There are additional requirements if an applicant fails an exam 3 or more times. (See Health Occupations Article, Section 14-307(g).)

Massachusetts
Requires FCVS

Number of attempts at Licensing Exam
3 attempts at USMLE Step 3 or COMLEX (See Board Regulations 243 CMR 2.02 (3)(b).)
Minimum Postgraduate Training Required
Prior to January 2014, 2 years for domestic graduates and 2 years for IMGs. After January 2014, 2 years for domestic graduates and 3 years for IMGs.
Time Limit for Completing Licensing Examination Sequence
7 years to complete USMLE or COMLEX. May request a waiver under specific conditions. (See Board Regulations 243 CMR 2.02 (3)(c)(2).)

Michigan Medical
Accepts FCVS
Number of attempts at Licensing Exam
3 attempts at each USMLE Step
Minimum Postgraduate Training Required
1 year
Time Limit for Completing Licensing Examination Sequence
Must pass all Steps of the USMLE within 7 years from the date of first passing any Step of the exam. Must pass Step 3 within 4 years of the first attempt at Step 3 or must complete 1 year of post-graduate training before making additional attempts at Step 3.

Michigan Osteopathic
Accepts FCVS
Number of attempts at Licensing Exam
6 attempts total for each examination
Minimum Postgraduate Training Required
1 year in AOA approved program
Time Limit for Completing Licensing Examination Sequence
Pass all components of the COMLEX-USA within 7 years from the date you first passed any component of the COMLEX-USA.

Minnesota
Accepts FCVS
Number of attempts at Licensing Exam
3 attempts at each USMLE Step,
4 attempts allowed if current license in another State and current certification by specialty board of ABMS, AOABPE, RCPSC, CFPC.
3 attempts at each COMLEX Level.
Minimum Postgraduate Training Required

1 year
Time Limit for Completing Licensing Examination Sequence
USMLE or COMLEX Step or Level 3 must be passed within 5 years of Step or Level 2 or before the end of residency training.

Mississippi
Accepts FCVS
Number of attempts at Licensing Exam
3 attempts at each Step
No limit on COMLEX
Minimum Postgraduate Training Required
1 year
1-3 years IMG
Time Limit for Completing Licensing Examination Sequence
7 years to complete USMLE
No limit on COMLEX

Missouri
Accepts FCVS
Number of attempts at Licensing Exam
3 attempts at USMLE Step 3
3 attempts on COMLEX
Minimum Postgraduate Training Required
1 year
3 years IMG
Time Limit for Completing Licensing Examination Sequence
7 years to complete USMLE (waived for MD/PhD candidates)
No limit on COMLEX

Montana
Accepts FCVS
Number of attempts at Licensing Exam
If an applicant fails to pass the first attempt at USMLE Step III, the applicant may be reexamined no more than five additional times.
No limit on COMLEX
Minimum Postgraduate Training Required
Completion of an approved residency program
3 years IMG
Time Limit for Completing Licensing Examination Sequence
7 years to complete USMLE (exceptions possible for MD/PhD candidates)

No limit on COMLEX.

Nebraska
Accepts FCVS
Number of attempts at Licensing Exam
4 attempts+ at each USMLE Step
4 attempts+ at each COMLEX Level
Minimum Postgraduate Training Required
1 year
2 years IMG
Time Limit for Completing Licensing Examination Sequence
10 years to complete USMLE or COMLEX beginning with date first Step/Level is passed.

Nevada Medical
Accepts FCVS
Number of attempts at Licensing Exam
Must pass all 3 Steps of USMLE in not more than a total of 9 attempts and must pass Step 3 in not more than a total of 3 attempts
Minimum Postgraduate Training Required
3 years. An unlimited license may be granted to currently enrolled residents in a post graduate training program in the U.S. or Canada, that have completed at least 24 months of progressive post graduate training and meet all requirements for an unlimited license in the state of Nevada, including having passed all 3 steps of USMLE within the time period allowed by NAC 630.080 and commit in writing to the Nevada State Board of Medical Examiners that they will complete the program and provide satisfactory completion of the program within 60 days after the scheduled completion of the program.
Time Limit for Completing Licensing Examination Sequence
MD must pass all Steps of the exam within 7 years after the date on which the applicant first passes any Step of the exam; PhD must pass all Steps of the exam within 10 years after the date on which the applicant first passes any Step of the exam.

Nevada Osteopathic
Requires FCVS
Number of attempts at Licensing Exam
No limit on COMLEX
Minimum Postgraduate Training Required
3 years for full license OR 2 years if resident signs commitment to practice in NV

Time Limit for Completing Licensing Examination Sequence
No limit on COMLEX

New Hampshire
Requires FCVS
Number of attempts at Licensing Exam
3 attempts at each USMLE Step or COMLEX Level
Minimum Postgraduate Training Required
2 years
Time Limit for Completing Licensing Examination Sequence
No limit on USMLE or COMLEX

New Jersey
Accepts FCVS
Number of attempts at Licensing Exam
5 attempts at USMLE Step 3
No information available on COMLEX
Minimum Postgraduate Training Required
US and IMG graduates who graduated after July 1, 2003 must complete 2 years of post-graduate training and have signed a contract for a 3rd
year in an accredited program. At least 2 of the years must be in the same field. Graduates prior to July 1, 2003: 1 year; 3 years IMG.
Time Limit for Completing Licensing Examination Sequence
7 years to complete USMLE
No information available on COMLEX

New Mexico Medical
Highly recommends FCVS
Number of attempts at Licensing Exam
6 attempts per USMLE Step
Minimum Postgraduate Training Required
2 years
Time Limit for Completing Licensing Examination Sequence
7 years to complete USMLE
10 years for MD/PhD candidates.

New Mexico Osteopathic
Highly recommends FCVS
Number of attempts at Licensing Exam
No limit on COMLEX

Minimum Postgraduate Training Required
1 year
Time Limit for Completing Licensing Examination Sequence
Within 7 years of having passed the first level

New York
Accepts FCVS for domestic graduates
IMGs-FCVS required
Number of attempts at Licensing Exam
No limit on USMLE or COMLEX
Minimum Postgraduate Training Required
Domestic 1 year
IMG 3 years
Time Limit for Completing Licensing Examination Sequence
No limit on USMLE or COMLEX

North Carolina
Accepts FCVS
Requires FCVS for Physicians with an established FCVS Profile and for IMG's (unless eligible for an Expedited License)
Number of attempts at Licensing Exam
3 attempts per USMLE Step
3 attempts per COMLEX Level
Minimum Postgraduate Training Required
1 year
2 years IMG
Time Limit for Completing Licensing Examination Sequence
No time limit for passing all 3 steps

North Dakota
Accepts FCVS
Number of attempts at Licensing Exam
3 attempts at each USMLE Step or COMLEX Level
Minimum Postgraduate Training Required
1 year
30 months IMG of ACGME accredited training
Time Limit for Completing Licensing Examination Sequence
7 years to complete USMLE or COMLEX

Northern Mariana Islands
Accepts FCVS
Number of attempts at Licensing Exam
No information available currently
Minimum Postgraduate Training Required
No information available currently
Time Limit for Completing Licensing Examination Sequence
No information available currently

Ohio
Requires FCVS
Number of attempts at Licensing Exam
Cannot have exceeded the maximum number of attempts for any step or level established by the NBME or NBOME, as effective on the date of application for a license. The board may grant a waiver if (1) the applicant holds current specialty board certification; or (2) demonstrates that a step or level was completed within the maximum number of attempts permitted by the NBME or NBOME at the time the step or level was successfully completed, provided that the applicant did not exceed six attempts for the step or level.
Minimum Postgraduate Training Required
1 year
2 years IMG
Time Limit for Completing Licensing Examination Sequence
10 years to complete USMLE or COMLEX (possible waiver good cause if over 10 years).

Oklahoma Medical
Accept FCVS
Number of attempts at Licensing Exam
3 attempts at each USMLE Step
(Step 2 = CK & CS)
Minimum Postgraduate Training Required
1 year
2 years IMG
Time Limit for Completing Licensing Examination Sequence
10 years to complete USMLE

Oklahoma Osteopathic
Accepts FCVS
Number of attempts at Licensing Exam

Contact the board for information
Minimum Postgraduate Training Required
1 year
Time Limit for Completing Licensing Examination Sequence
No limit on COMLEX

Oregon
Accepts FCVS
Number of attempts at Licensing Exam
3 attempts at USMLE step 3/COMLEX level 3. 4th attempt after additional 1 year post graduate training. Waiver of attempt requirement may be available if ABMS/AOA certified.
Minimum Postgraduate Training Required
1 year
3 years IMG
Time Limit for Completing Licensing Examination Sequence
7 years to complete USMLE or COMLEX

Pennsylvania Medical
Accepts FCVS
Number of attempts at Licensing Exam
No more than 4 attempts at each Step or Step Component
Minimum Postgraduate Training Required
2 years
Time Limit for Completing Licensing Examination Sequence
No time limit

Pennsylvania Osteopathic
Accepts FCVS
Number of attempts at Licensing Exam
No limit on COMLEX
Minimum Postgraduate Training Required
1 year
Time Limit for Completing Licensing Examination Sequence
No limit on COMLEX

Puerto Rico
Accepts FCVS
Number of attempts at Licensing Exam
No limit on USMLE
Minimum Postgraduate Training Required

1 year
Time Limit for Completing Licensing Examination Sequence
USMLE Step 3 shall be passed within 7 years of the date of passing Step 1.

Rhode Island
Requires FCVS
Number of attempts at Licensing Exam
3 attempts at each USMLE Step
3 attempts at each COMLEX Level
Minimum Postgraduate Training Required
2 years
2 years IMG
Time Limit for Completing Licensing Examination Sequence
No time limit

American Samoa
Number of attempts at Licensing Exam
No information available currently
Minimum Postgraduate Training Required
No information available currently
Time Limit for Completing Licensing Examination Sequence
No information available currently

South Carolina
Requires FCVS
Number of attempts at Licensing Exam
4 attempts per USMLE Step and COMLEX Level
Minimum Postgraduate Training Required
1 year
3 years IMG
Time Limit for Completing Licensing Examination Sequence
10 years to complete USMLE or COMLEX

South Dakota
Accepts FCVS
Number of attempts at Licensing Exam
Allowed 3 attempts, must pass on third, for the USMLE or COMLEX examination
Minimum Postgraduate Training Required
Successful completion of residency program
Time Limit for Completing Licensing Examination Sequence

7 years to complete USMLE or COMLEX
10 years for Dual Program Degree MD-PhD Applicant

Tennessee Medical
Accepts FCVS
Number of attempts at Licensing Exam
If an applicant fails any step of the USMLE or FLEX examinations more than four (4) times, then the Board shall require proof of board-certification by an ABMS-recognized specialty board and proof of meeting requirements for Maintenance of Certification prior to application before consideration for licensure.
Minimum Postgraduate Training Required
1 year
3 years IMG
Time Limit for Completing Licensing Examination Sequence
All three steps must be taken and passed within ten (10) years of the first successful step, unless you qualify under an exception.
Tennessee Osteopathic Accepts FCVS
Number of attempts at Licensing Exam
3 attempts
Minimum Postgraduate Training Required
1 year
Time Limit for Completing Licensing Examination Sequence
No limit on COMLEX

Texas
Accepts FCVS
Number of attempts at Licensing Exam
3 attempts at each USMLE Step or COMLEX Level. (Exceptions may apply for applicants who held a Texas Physician in Training permit on or before September 1, 2005 or who have been licensed in good standing in another state for 5 years. See
TMB website
for more information,)
Minimum Postgraduate Training Required
1 year
2 years IMG
Time Limit for Completing Licensing Examination Sequence
7 years+ to complete the USMLE or COMLEX. (Exceptions may apply for applicants who are especially board certified or who completed combined MD/PhD programs, or who exceed the time limit but are willing to accept a

limited license to practice exclusively in an MUA or HPSA. See TMB website for more information.)

Utah Medical
Requires FCVS
Number of attempts at Licensing Exam
3 attempts at each USMLE Step or COMLEX Level
Minimum Postgraduate Training Required
1 year
2 years IMG
Time Limit for Completing Licensing Examination Sequence
7 years+
to complete the USMLE or COMLEX
10 years for MD/PhD candidates or DO/PhD candidates

Vermont Medical
Accepts FCVS
Number of attempts at Licensing Exam
3 attempts at USMLE Step 3
Minimum Postgraduate Training Required
2 years
3 years IMG
Time Limit for Completing Licensing Examination Sequence
7 years to complete USMLE

Vermont Osteopathic
Accepts FCVS
Number of attempts at Licensing Exam
No information available currently
Minimum Postgraduate Training Required
1-year rotating internship or 3-year residency program
Time Limit for Completing Licensing Examination Sequence
No information available currently

Virgin Islands
Requires FCVS
Number of attempts at Licensing Exam
Must take SPEX (only given in May and November) and an oral exam. 2 attempts
Minimum Postgraduate Training Required
6 months required after 2 attempts for SPEX exam

Virginia
Accepts FCVS
Number of attempts at Licensing Exam
4 attempts on any USMLE step with a 5th attempt considered upon petition or appeal submitted to the Board to be reviewed in accordance with Board policy in
Minimum Postgraduate Training Required
1 year
Time Limit for Completing Licensing Examination Sequence
10 years to complete USMLE; Greater than 10 years if candidate is ABMS certified.

Washington Medical
Accepts FCVS
Number of attempts at Licensing Exam
3 attempts at USMLE Step 3
Minimum Postgraduate Training Required
2 years
Time Limit for Completing Licensing Examination Sequence
7 years+ to complete USMLE

Washington Osteopathic
Accepts FCVS
Number of attempts at Licensing Exam
3 attempts on COMLEX
Minimum Postgraduate Training Required
1 year
Time Limit for Completing Licensing Examination Sequence
No limit on COMLEX

West Virginia Medical
Accepts FCVS
Number of attempts at Licensing Exam
6 attempts per USMLE Step or Step component
Minimum Postgraduate Training Required
1 year
3 years IMG

Time Limit for Completing Licensing Examination Sequence
10 years to complete USMLE

West Virginia Osteopathic
Accepts FCVS
Number of attempts at Licensing Exam
No limit on COMLEX
Minimum Postgraduate Training Required
1 year
Time Limit for Completing Licensing Examination Sequence
No limit on COMLEX

Wisconsin
Accepts FCVS
Number of attempts at Licensing Exam
3 attempts at each USMLE step/COMLEX level
Minimum Postgraduate Training Required
2 years
Time Limit for Completing Licensing Examination Sequence
USMLE Step 3 shall be passed within 10 years of the date of passing Step 1
N/A on COMLEX.

Wyoming
Requires FCVS
Number of attempts at Licensing Exam
7 total attempts on USMLE or COMLEX in 7 years
Minimum Postgraduate Training Required
2 years (1 year if applicant has current certification by an ABMS or AOABOS/BOC specialty board, or continuous licensure in good standing in 1 or more states and/or D.C. for the preceding 5 years.)
Time Limit for Completing Licensing Examination Sequence
7 years (8 years if in combined DO or MD/PhD program)

--END OF LIST--

APPENDIX Di

RESIDENCY PROGRAMS BY STATE
SURGERY – GENERAL

APPENDIX Di

RESIDENCY PROGRAMS BY STATE
SURGERY - GENERAL

Please visit AMA/FREIDA online for detailed and up to date information on programs.
https://freida.ama-assn.org
The following information is provided based on free online resources and program websites.

SURGERY-GENERAL
University of Alabama Medical Center Program
Birmingham, AL

Brookwood Baptist Health Program
Birmingham, AL

USA Health Program
Mobile, AL

University of Arkansas for Medical Sciences (UAMS) College of Medicine Program
Little Rock, AR

Dignity Health East Valley Program
Chandler, AZ

Abrazo Health Network Program
Glendale, AZ

Midwestern University GME Consortium/Mountain Vista Program
Mesa, AZ

HonorHealth Program
Phoenix, AZ

Mayo Clinic College of Medicine and Science (Phoenix) Program
Phoenix, AZ

University of Arizona College of Medicine-Phoenix Program
Phoenix, AZ

Creighton University School of Medicine Program
Phoenix, AZ

University of Arizona College of Medicine-Tucson Program
Tucson, AZ

Kern Medical Center Program
Bakersfield, CA

Arrowhead Regional Medical Center/Kaiser Permanente (Fontana) Program
Colton, CA

San Joaquin General Hospital Program
French Camp, CA

University of California (San Francisco)/Fresno Program
Fresno, CA

University of California (San Diego) Medical Center Program
La Jolla, CA

Loma Linda University Health Education Consortium Program
Loma Linda, CA

Cedars-Sinai Medical Center Program
Los Angeles, CA

University of Southern California/Los Angeles General Medical Center (USC/LA General) Program
Los Angeles, CA

Kaiser Permanente Southern California (Los Angeles) Program
Los Angeles, CA

UCLA David Geffen School of Medicine/UCLA Medical Center Program
Los Angeles, CA

Riverside University Health System/University of California Riverside Program
Moreno Valley, CA

University of California San Francisco (East Bay) Program
Oakland, CA

University of California (Irvine) Program
Orange, CA

Desert Regional Medical Center Program
Palm Springs, CA

Huntington Memorial Hospital Program
Pasadena, CA

HCA Healthcare Riverside Program
Riverside, CA

Sutter Health/Sutter Roseville Medical Center Program
Roseville, CA

University of California Davis Health Program
Sacramento, CA

Naval Medical Center (San Diego) Program
San Diego, CA

University of California (San Francisco) Program
San Francisco, CA

Santa Barbara Cottage Hospital Program
Santa Barbara, CA

Stanford Health Care-Sponsored Stanford University Program
Stanford, CA

HCA Healthcare/Los Robles Regional Medical Center Program
Thousand Oaks, CA

Los Angeles County-Harbor-UCLA Medical Center Program
Torrance, CA

Community Memorial Health System Program
Ventura, CA

Kaweah Delta Health Care District (KDHCD) Program
Visalia, CA

Southwest Healthcare Medical Education Consortium Program
Wildomar, CA

University of Colorado Program
Aurora, CO

Saint Joseph Hospital Program
Denver, CO

HCA Health One/Swedish Medical Center Program
Englewood, CO

Kansas City University GME Consortium (KCU-GME Consortium)/St Anthony Program
Lakewood, CO

HCA Health One/Sky Ridge Medical Center Program
Lone Tree, CO

Danbury Hospital Program
Danbury, CT

University of Connecticut Program
Farmington, CT

Yale-New Haven Medical Center Program
New Haven, CT

Stamford Hospital/Columbia University College of Physicians and Surgeons Program
Stamford, CT

Quinnipiac University Frank H Netter MD School of Medicine(Waterbury Hospital) Program
Waterbury, CT

St Mary's Hospital (Waterbury) Program
Waterbury, CT

MedStar Health/Georgetown-Washington Hospital Program
Washington, DC

George Washington University Program
Washington, DC

Howard University Program
Washington, DC

Bayhealth Medical Center Program
Dover, DE
ID: 4400900001

Christiana Care Health Services Program
Newark, DE

HCA Florida JFK Hospital/University of Miami Miller School of Medicine GME Consortium Program
Atlantis, FL

Florida Atlantic University Charles E Schmidt College of Medicine Program
Boca Raton, FL

HCA Florida Healthcare/USF Morsani College of Medicine GME Brandon Hospital Program
Brandon, FL

Broward Health Program
Fort Lauderdale, FL

University of Miami Hospital and Clinics Program
Fort Lauderdale, FL

HCA Florida Healthcare/Lawnwood Hospital Program
Fort Pierce, FL

University of Florida Program
Gainesville, FL

HCA Florida Healthcare/USF Morsani College of Medicine GME Bayonet Point Hospital Program
Hudson, FL

University of Florida College of Medicine Jacksonville Program
Jacksonville, FL

Mayo Clinic College of Medicine and Science (Jacksonville) Program
Jacksonville, FL

Lakeland Regional Health Program
Lakeland, FL

University of Miami/Jackson Health System Program
Miami, FL

HCA Florida Healthcare/Kendall Hospital Program
Miami, FL

Florida International University / Baptist Health Program
Miami, FL

Mount Sinai Medical Center of Florida Program
Miami Beach, FL

University of Central Florida/HCA Florida Healthcare (Ocala) Program
Ocala, FL

HCA Florida Orange Park Hospital Program
Orange Park, FL

University of Central Florida/HCA Florida Healthcare (Greater Orlando/Osceola) Program
Orlando, FL

Orlando Health Program
Orlando, FL

Advent Health Florida (Orlando) Program
Orlando, FL

Memorial Healthcare System (Hollywood Florida) Program
Pembroke Pines, FL

University of Central Florida/HCA Florida Healthcare (Pensacola) Program
Pensacola, FL

HCA Florida Healthcare/Westside/Northwest Hospital Program
Plantation, FL

Larkin Community Hospital Program
South Miami, FL

Florida State University College of Medicine Program
Tallahassee, FL

Advent Health Florida (Tampa) Program
Tampa, FL

BayCare Health System Program
Tampa, FL

University of South Florida Morsani Program
Tampa, FL

Cleveland Clinic (Florida) Program
Weston, FL

Emory University School of Medicine Program
Atlanta, GA

Morehouse School of Medicine Program
Atlanta, GA

Medical College of Georgia Program
Augusta, GA

Dwight David Eisenhower Army Medical Center Program
Fort Gordon, GA

Northeast Georgia Medical Center Program
Gainesville, GA

Atrium Health Navicent The Medical Center/Mercer University School of Medicine Program
Macon, GA

Wellstar Health System/Wellstar Kennestone Regional Medical Center Program
Marietta, GA

HCA Healthcare/Mercer University School of Medicine/Memorial Health-University Medical Center Program
Savannah, GA

University of Hawaii Program
Honolulu, HI

Tripler Army Medical Center Program
Tripler AMC, HI

Mercy One Des Moines/PHC Consortium Program
Des Moines, IA

Central Iowa Health System (Iowa Methodist Medical Center)Program
Des Moines, IA

University of Iowa Hospitals and Clinics Program
Iowa City, IA

University of Chicago Program
Chicago, IL

McGaw Medical Center of Northwestern University Program
Chicago, IL

Rush University Medical Center Program
Chicago, IL

University of Illinois College of Medicine at Chicago (Mount Sinai) Program
Chicago, IL

University of Illinois College of Medicine at Chicago Program
Chicago, IL

Ascension Illinois/Saint Joseph (Chicago) Program
Chicago, IL

University of Illinois College of Medicine at Chicago (Metropolitan Group) Program
Chicago, IL

Loyola University Medical Center Program
Maywood, IL

Franciscan Health Olympia Fields Program
Olympia Fields, IL

Advocate Health Care Program
Park Ridge, IL

University of Illinois College of Medicine at Peoria Program
Peoria, IL

Southern Illinois University Program
Springfield, IL

Carle Foundation Hospital Program
Urbana, IL

Parkview Health Program
Fort Wayne, IN

Ascension St Vincent Hospital Indianapolis Program
Indianapolis, IN

Indiana University School of Medicine Program
Indianapolis, IN

University of Kansas School of Medicine Program
Kansas City, KS

HCA Healthcare Kansas City/Menorah Medical Center Program
Overland Park, KS

University of Kansas (Wichita) Program
Wichita, KS

University of Kentucky College of Medicine (Bowling Green) Program
Bowling Green, KY

University of Kentucky College of Medicine Program
Lexington, KY

University of Louisville School of Medicine Program
Louisville, KY

Ochsner Lafayette General Medical Center Program
Lafayette, LA

Louisiana State University School of Medicine Program
New Orleans, LA

Tulane University Program
New Orleans, LA

Ochsner Clinic Foundation Program
New Orleans, LA

Willis-Knighton Health System Program
Shreveport, LA

Louisiana State University (Shreveport) Program
Shreveport, LA

Boston University Medical Center Program
Boston, MA

Tufts Medical Center Program
Boston, MA

Mass General Brigham/Brigham and Women's Hospital Program
Boston, MA

Mass General Brigham/Massachusetts General Hospital Program
Boston, MA

Beth Israel Deaconess Medical Center Program
Boston, MA

St Elizabeth's Medical Center Program
Brighton, MA

Lahey Clinic Program
Burlington, MA

Berkshire Medical Center Program
Pittsfield, MA

UMass Chan-Baystate Program
Springfield, MA

UMass Chan Medical School Program
Worcester, MA

Anne Arundel Medical Center Program
Annapolis, MD

MedStar Health (Baltimore) Program
Baltimore, MD

University of Maryland Program
Baltimore, MD

Johns Hopkins University Program
Baltimore, MD

Sinai Hospital of Baltimore Program
Baltimore, MD

St Agnes HealthCare Program
Baltimore, MD

National Capital Consortium Program
Bethesda, MD

Tidal Health Program
Salisbury, MD

Maine Medical Center (Rural Track) Program
Portland, ME

Maine Health Program
Portland, ME

University of Michigan Program
Ann Arbor, MI

Henry Ford Health/Henry Ford Macomb Hospital Program
Clinton Township, MI

Corewell Health (Dearborn and Trenton) Program
Dearborn, MI

Detroit Medical Center Corporation Program
Detroit, MI

Ascension St John Hospital Program
Detroit, MI

Detroit Medical Center/Wayne State University Program
Detroit, MI

Detroit Medical Center Corporation Program
Detroit, MI

Corewell Health (Farmington Hills) Program
Farmington Hills, MI

Garden City Hospital Program
Garden City, MI

Ascension Genesys Hospital Program
Grand Blanc, MI

Corewell Health-Grand Rapids/Michigan State University Program
Grand Rapids, MI

Henry Ford Health/Henry Ford Jackson Hospital Program
Jackson, MI

Western Michigan University Homer Stryker MD School ofMedicine Program
Kalamazoo, MI

University of Michigan Health - Sparrow Program
Lansing, MI

McLaren Health Care/Greater Lansing/MSU Program
Lansing, MI

McLaren Health Care/Macomb/MSU Program
Mount Clemens, MI

Trinity Health Oakland/Wayne State University Program
Pontiac, MI

Corewell Health (Royal Oak) Program
Royal Oak, MI

Central Michigan University College of Medicine/CMU Medical Education Partners Program
Saginaw, MI

Ascension Providence/MSUCHM Program
Southfield, MI

Ascension Macomb-Oakland Hospital Program
Warren, MI

Henry Ford Health/Henry Ford Wyandotte Hospital Program
Wyandotte, MI

University of Michigan Health-West Program
Wyoming, MI

Trinity Health Ann Arbor Hospital Program
Ypsilanti, MI

Hennepin Healthcare Program
Minneapolis, MN

University of Minnesota Program
Minneapolis, MN

Mayo Clinic College of Medicine and Science (Rochester) Program
Rochester, MN

Kansas City University GME Consortium (KCU-GME Consortium)/St Mary's Program
Blue Springs, MO

University of Missouri-Columbia Program
Columbia, MO

University of Missouri-Kansas City School of Medicine Program
Kansas City, MO

Washington University/B-JH/SLCH Consortium Program
Saint Louis, MO

SSM Health/Saint Louis University School of Medicine Program
St Louis, MO

University of Mississippi Medical Center Program
Jackson, MS

Keesler Medical Center Program
Keesler AFB, MS

Mountain Area Health Education Center Program
Asheville, NC

University of North Carolina Hospitals Program
Chapel Hill, NC

Carolinas Medical Center Program
Charlotte, NC

Duke University Hospital Program
Durham, NC

Cape Fear Valley Health Program
Fayetteville, NC

Womack Army Medical Center Program
Fort Liberty, NC

ECU Health Medical Center/East Carolina University Program
Greenville, NC

Novant Health New Hanover Regional Medical Center Program
Wilmington, NC

Wake Forest University Baptist Medical Center Program
Winston-Salem, NC

University of North Dakota Program
Grand Forks, ND

University of Nebraska Medical Center College of Medicine Program
Omaha, NE

Creighton University School of Medicine (Omaha) Program
Omaha, NE

Dartmouth-Hitchcock/Mary Hitchcock Memorial Hospital Program
Lebanon, NH

Care Point Health/Bayonne Medical Center Program
Bayonne, NJ

Virtua Program
Camden, NJ

Cooper Medical School of Rowan University/Cooper University Hospital Program
Camden, NJ

Hackensack University Medical Center Program
Hackensack, NJ

Rutgers Health/Monmouth Medical Center Program
Long Branch, NJ

Atlantic Health System/Morristown Medical Center Program
Morristown, NJ

Inspira Health Network/Inspira Medical Center Vineland Program
Mullica Hill, NJ

Jersey Shore University Medical Center Program
Neptune, NJ

Rutgers Health/Robert Wood Johnson Medical School Program
New Brunswick, NJ

Rutgers Health/New Jersey Medical School Program
Newark, NJ

Hackensack University Medical Center (Palisades) Program
North Bergen, NJ

Icahn School of Medicine at Mount Sinai Program
Paramus, NJ

St Joseph's University Medical Center Program
Paterson, NJ

Holy Name Medical Center Program
Teaneck, NJ

Rutgers Health/Community Medical Center Program
Toms River, NJ

University of New Mexico School of Medicine Program
Albuquerque, NM

Valley Health System Program
Las Vegas, NV

Kirk Kerkorian School of Medicine at UNLV Program
Las Vegas, NV

HCA Healthcare Sunrise Health GME/Mountain View Program
Las Vegas, NV

Albany Medical Center Program
Albany, NY

Zucker School of Medicine at Hofstra/Northwell at South Shore University Hospital Program
Bayshore, NY

Montefiore Medical Center/Albert Einstein College of Medicine Program
Bronx, NY

Lincoln Medical and Mental Health Center Program
Bronx, NY

St Barnabas Hospital Program
Bronx, NY

BronxCare Health System Program
Bronx, NY

One Brooklyn Health System/Brookdale University Hospital and Medical Center Program
Brooklyn, NY

NYC Health & Hospitals/South Brooklyn Health Program
Brooklyn, NY

Maimonides Medical Center Program
Brooklyn, NY

New York-Presbyterian Brooklyn Methodist Hospital Program
Brooklyn, NY

SUNY Downstate Health Sciences University Program
Brooklyn, NY

Brooklyn Hospital Center Program
Brooklyn, NY

Wyckoff Heights Medical Center Program
Brooklyn, NY

NYU Grossman School of Medicine (Brooklyn) Program
Brooklyn, NY

University at Buffalo Program
Buffalo, NY

Bassett Medical Center Program
Cooperstown, NY

Nassau University Medical Center Program
East Meadow, NY

St John's Episcopal Hospital-South Shore Program
Far Rockaway, NY

Flushing Hospital Medical Center Program
Flushing, NY

New York-Presbyterian/Queens Program
Flushing, NY

Zucker School of Medicine at Hofstra/Northwell Program
Manhasset, NY

Garnet Health Medical Center Program
Middletown, NY

NYU Grossman Long Island School of Medicine Program
Mineola, NY

New York Presbyterian Hospital (Cornell Campus) Program
New York, NY

New York Presbyterian Hospital (Columbia Campus) Program
New York, NY

NYU Grossman School of Medicine Program
New York, NY

New York Medical College at Metropolitan Hospital Center Program
New York, NY

Icahn School of Medicine at Mount Sinai Program
New York, NY
Harlem Hospital Center Program
New York, NY

Zucker School of Medicine at Hofstra/Northwell at Lenox Hill Hospital Program
New York, NY

Icahn School of Medicine at Mount Sinai/South Nassau Program
Oceanside, NY

Nuvance Health Program
Poughkeepsie, NY

University of Rochester Program
Rochester, NY

Good Samaritan University Hospital/St Catherine of Siena Hospital Program
Smithtown, NY

Stony Brook Medicine/Southampton Hospital Program
Southampton, NY

Zucker School of Medicine at Hofstra/Northwell at Staten Island University Hospital Program
Staten Island, NY

Stony Brook Medicine Program
Stony Brook, NY

SUNY Upstate Medical University Program
Syracuse, NY

Mohawk Valley Health System, Inc Program
Utica, NY

Westchester Medical Center Program
Valhalla, NY

Akron General Medical Center/NEOMED Program
Akron, OH

Summa Health System/NEOMED Program
Akron, OH

University of Cincinnati Medical Center/College of Medicine Program
Cincinnati, OH

TriHealth (Good Samaritan Hospital) Program
Cincinnati, OH

Jewish Hospital of Cincinnati Program
Cincinnati, OH

The MetroHealth System/Case Western Reserve University Program
Cleveland, OH

Case Western Reserve University/University Hospitals Cleveland Medical Center Program
Cleveland, OH

Cleveland Clinic Foundation Program
Cleveland, OH

OhioHealth/Doctors Hospital Program
Columbus, OH

OhioHealth/Riverside Methodist Hospital Program
Columbus, OH

Ohio State University Hospital Program
Columbus, OH

Western Reserve Hospital Program
Cuyahoga Falls, OH

Kettering Health Network Program
Dayton, OH

Wright State University Program
Dayton, OH

Mount Carmel Health System Program
Grove City, OH

Mercy St Vincent Medical Center Program
Toledo, OH

University of Toledo Program
Toledo, OH

Western Reserve Health Education/NEOMED Program
Warren, OH

Cleveland Clinic Foundation/South Pointe Hospital Program
Warrensville Heights, OH

St Elizabeth Youngstown Hospital/NEOMED Program
Youngstown, OH

University of Oklahoma Health Sciences Center Program
Oklahoma City, OK

Oklahoma State University Center for Health Sciences Program
Tulsa, OK

University of Oklahoma School of Community Medicine (Tulsa)Program
Tulsa, OK

Samaritan Health Services-Corvallis Program
Corvallis, OR

Oregon Health & Science University (OHSU Health) Program
Portland, OR

Abington Memorial Hospital Program
Abington, PA

Lehigh Valley Health Network Program
Allentown, PA

St Luke's University Hospital Program
Bethlehem, PA

Geisinger Health System Program
Danville, PA

Mercy Catholic Medical Center Program
Darby, PA

UPMC Medical Education (Farrell) Program
Farrell, PA

UPMC Medical Education (Harrisburg) Community Program
Harrisburg, PA

UPMC Medical Education (Harrisburg) Program
Harrisburg, PA

UPMC Medical Education Program
Harrisburg, PA

Medical Center Program
Hershey, PA

Conemaugh Memorial Medical Center Program
Johnstown, PA

Philadelphia College of Osteopathic Medicine Program
Philadelphia, PA

Jefferson Health Medical Education/Jefferson Einstein Philadelphia Hospital Program
Philadelphia, PA

Nazareth Hospital Program
Philadelphia, PA

Temple University Hospital Program
Philadelphia, PA

Sidney Kimmel Medical College at Thomas Jefferson University/TJUH Program
Philadelphia, PA

University of Pennsylvania Health System Program
Philadelphia, PA

Allegheny Health Network Medical Education Consortium (AGH)Program
Pittsburgh, PA

UPMC Medical Education/Mercy Program
Pittsburgh, PA

UPMC Medical Education (Pittsburgh) Program
Pittsburgh, PA

Robert Packer Hospital/Guthrie Program
Sayre, PA

Tower Health Program
West Reading, PA

Geisinger Health System (Wilkes Barre) Program
Wilkes-Barre, PA

Main Line Health System/Lankenau Medical Center Program
Wynnewood, PA

Wellspan Health/York Hospital Program
York, PA

Hospital Episcopal San Lucas/Ponce School of Medicine Program
Ponce, PR

University of Puerto Rico Program
San Juan, PR

Brown University Program
Providence, RI

HCA Healthcare/Mercer University School of Medicine/Trident Medical Center Program
Charleston, SC

Medical University of South Carolina Program
Charleston, SC

Prisma Health/University of South Carolina School of Medicine Columbia (Columbia) Program
Columbia, SC

Prisma Health/University of South Carolina School of Medicine Greenville (Greenville) Program
Greenville, SC

HCA Healthcare/Mercer University School of Medicine/Grand Strand Medical Center Program
Myrtle Beach, SC

Spartanburg Medical Center Program
Spartanburg, SC

University of South Dakota School of Medicine Program
Sioux Falls, SD

University of Tennessee College of Medicine at Chattanooga Program
Chattanooga, TN

East Tennessee State University/Quillen College of Medicine Program
Johnson City, TN

University of Tennessee Medical Center at Knoxville Program
Knoxville, TN

University of Tennessee Program
Memphis, TN

Baptist Memorial Medical Education Program
Memphis, TN

University of Tennessee College of Medicine (Nashville) Program
Nashville, TN

Vanderbilt University Medical Center Program
Nashville, TN

Texas Tech University Health Sciences Center at Amarillo Program
Amarillo, TX

University of Texas at Austin Dell Medical School Program
Austin, TX

St David's Healthcare Graduate Medical Education Program
Austin, TX

Methodist Health System Dallas Program
Dallas, TX

Baylor University Medical Center Program
Dallas, TX

University of Texas Southwestern Medical Center Program
Dallas, TX

Doctors Hospital at Renaissance Ltd Program
Edinburg, TX

Texas Tech University HSC El Paso Program
El Paso, TX

William Beaumont Army Medical Center Program
El Paso, TX

Baylor All Saints Medical Center Fort Worth Program
Fort Worth, TX

Texas Health Resources Fort Worth General Surgery Program
Fort Worth, TX

University of Texas Medical Branch Hospitals Program
Galveston, TX

University of Texas Rio Grande Valley Program
Harlingen, TX

Baylor College of Medicine Program
Houston, TX

University of Texas Health Science Center at Houston Program
Houston, TX

Methodist Hospital (Houston) Program
Houston, TX

San Antonio Uniformed Services Health Education Consortium Program
JBSA Ft Sam Houston, TX

HCA Houston Healthcare/University of Houston (Kingwood)Program
Kingwood, TX

Texas Tech University Health Sciences Center at Lubbock Program
Lubbock, TX

Texas Tech University Health Sciences Center (Permian Basin) Program
Odessa, TX

HCA Medical City Healthcare UNT-TCU GME (Plano) Program
Plano, TX

University of Texas Health Science Center San Antonio Joe and Teresa Lozano Long School of Medicine Program
San Antonio, TX

Methodist Healthcare System of San Antonio Program
San Antonio, TX

Texas A&M College of Medicine-Scott and White Medical Center(Temple) Program
Temple, TX

University of Texas Health Science Center at Tyler Program
Tyler, TX

HCA Houston Healthcare/University of Houston Program
Webster, TX

Intermountain Medical Center Program
Murray, UT

University of Utah Health Program
Salt Lake City, UT

University of Virginia Medical Center Program
Charlottesville, VA

Inova Fairfax Medical Campus/Inova Fairfax Hospital for Children Program
Falls Church, VA

Mary Washington Healthcare Program
Fredericksburg, VA

Eastern Virginia Medical School at Old Dominion University Program
Norfolk, VA

Naval Medical Center (Portsmouth) Program
Portsmouth, VA

Virginia Commonwealth University Health System Program
Richmond, VA

HCA Healthcare Chippenham & Johnston-Willis Hospitals Program
Richmond, VA

Carilion Clinic-Virginia Tech Carilion School of Medicine Program
Roanoke, VA

University of Vermont Medical Center Program
Burlington, VT

Virginia Mason Franciscan Health Program
Seattle, WA

University of Washington Program
Seattle, WA

Swedish Medical Center/First Hill Program
Seattle, WA

Virginia Mason Franciscan Health/St Joseph's Hospital Program
Tacoma, WA

Madigan Army Medical Center Program
Tacoma, WA

Gundersen Lutheran Medical Foundation Program
La Crosse, WI

University of Wisconsin Hospitals and Clinics Program
Madison, WI

Marshfield Clinic Program
Marshfield, WI

Medical College of Wisconsin Affiliated Hospitals Program
Milwaukee, WI

Charleston Area Medical Center/CAMC Institute for Academic Medicine Program
Charleston, WV

Marshall University School of Medicine Program
Huntington, WV

Marshall Community Health Consortium Program
Huntington, WV

West Virginia University Program
Morgantown, WV

APPENDIX Dii

RESIDENCY PROGRAMS BY STATE

PHYSICAL MEDICINE AND REHABILITATION

APPENDIX Dii

RESIDENCY PROGRAMS BY STATE
PHYSICAL MEDICINE AND REHABILITATION

PHYSICAL MEDICINE AND REHABILITATION
Please visit AMA/FREIDA online for detailed and up to date information on programs.
https://freida.ama-assn.org
The following information is provided based on free online resources and program websites.

University of Alabama Medical Center Program
Birmingham, AL

University of Arkansas for Medical Sciences (UAMS) College of Medicine Program
Little Rock, AR

Honor Health Program
Scottsdale, AZ

Loma Linda University Health Education Consortium Program
Loma Linda, CA

Charles R Drew University of Medicine and Science, College of Medicine Program
Los Angeles, CA

UCLA David Geffen School of Medicine/UCLA Medical Center/VA Greater Los Angeles Healthcare System Program
Los Angeles, CA

University of California (Irvine) Program
Orange, CA

OPTI West Program
Pomona, CA

Stanford Health Care-Sponsored Stanford University Program
Redwood City, CA

University of California Davis Health Program
Sacramento, CA

University of Colorado Program
Aurora, CO

University of Connecticut School of Medicine Program
Hartford, CT

Yale-New Haven Hospital Program
New Haven, CT

MedStar Health/Georgetown-National Rehabilitation Hospital Program
Washington, DC

HCA Florida Healthcare/USF Morsani College of Medicine GME Program
Bradenton, FL

Broward Health Program
Deerfield Bch, FL

University of Florida College of Medicine Program
Gainesville, FL

Larkin Community Hospital Palm Springs Campus Program
Hialeah, FL

Memorial Healthcare System (Hollywood Florida) Program
Hollywood, FL

Mayo Clinic College of Medicine and Science/Brooks Rehabilitation Hospital (Jacksonville) Program

University of Miami/Jackson Health System Program
Miami, FL

University of Central Florida/HCA Florida Healthcare (Pensacola)Program
Pensacola, FL

Larkin Community Hospital Program
South Miami, FL

University of South Florida Morsani (James A Haley Veterans Hospital) Program
Tampa, FL

Emory University School of Medicine Program
Atlanta, GA

McGaw Medical Center of Northwestern University Program
Chicago, IL

Rush University Medical Center Program
Chicago, IL

Schwab Rehabilitation Hospital and Care Network/University of Chicago Program
Chicago, IL

Northwestern Medicine Marianjoy Rehabilitation Hospital Program
Wheaton, IL

Parkview Health Program
Fort Wayne, IN

Indiana University School of Medicine Program
Indianapolis, IN

University of Kansas School of Medicine Program
Kansas City, KS

University of Kentucky College of Medicine Program
Lexington, KY

University of Louisville School of Medicine Program
Louisville, KY

Louisiana State University School of Medicine Program
New Orleans, LA

Tufts Medical Center Program
Boston, MA

Mass General Brigham/Spaulding Rehabilitation Hospital/Harvard Medical School Program
Charlestown, MA

Johns Hopkins University Program
Baltimore, MD

Sinai Hospital of Baltimore Program
Baltimore, MD

National Capital Consortium Program
Bethesda, ID: 3401021074

University of Michigan Program
Ann Arbor, MI

Detroit Medical Center/Wayne State University Program
Detroit, MI

University of Michigan Health - Sparrow/Michigan State University Program
East Lansing, MI

Mary Free Bed Hospital Program
Grand Rapids, MI

Corewell Health (Royal Oak) Program
Royal Oak, MI

Corewell Health (Taylor) Program
Taylor, MI

University of Minnesota Program
Minneapolis, MN

Mayo Clinic College of Medicine and Science (Rochester) Program
Rochester, MN

University of Missouri-Columbia Program
Columbia, MO

Washington University/B-JH/SLCH Consortium Program
St Louis, MO

University of North Carolina Hospitals Program
Chapel Hill, NC

Carolinas Medical Center Program
Charlotte, NC

ECU Health Medical Center/East Carolina University Program
Greenville, NC

University of Nebraska Medical Center College of Medicine Program
Omaha, NE

JFK Medical Center Program
Edison, NJ

Inspira Health Network Program
Mullica Hill, NJ

Rutgers Health/New Jersey Medical School Program
Newark, NJ

University of New Mexico School of Medicine Program
Albuquerque, NM

HCA Healthcare Sunrise Health GME/Mountain View Program
Las Vegas, NV

Albany Medical Center Program
Albany, NY

Montefiore Medical Center/Albert Einstein College of Medicine Program
Bronx, NY

SUNY Downstate Health Sciences University Program
Brooklyn, NY

One Brooklyn Health System/Kingsbrook Jewish Medical Center Program
Brooklyn, NY

Nassau University Medical Center Program
East Meadow, NY

Zucker School of Medicine at Hofstra/Northwell Program
Manhasset, NY

New York Presbyterian Hospital (Columbia and Cornell Campus) Program
New York, NY

Icahn School of Medicine at Mount Sinai Program
New York, NY

New York Medical College (Metropolitan) Program
New York, NY

NYU Grossman School of Medicine Program
New York, NY

Stony Brook Medicine/University Hospital Program
Port Jefferson, NY

University of Rochester Program
Rochester, NY

Rochester Regional Health/Unity Hospital Program
Rochester, NY

Good Samaritan University Hospital/Mercy Hospital Program
Rockville Centre, NY

SUNY Upstate Medical University Program
Syracuse, NY

Westchester Medical Center Program
Valhalla, NY

Burke Rehabilitation Hospital Program
White Plains, NY

University Hospitals Community Consortium Program
Chardon, OH

University of Cincinnati Medical Center/College of Medicine Program
Cincinnati, OH

Cleveland Clinic Foundation Program
Cleveland, OH

The Metro Health System/Case Western Reserve University Program
Cleveland, OH

Ohio State University Hospital Program
Columbus, OH

University of Toledo Program
Toledo, OH

Geisinger Health System Program
Bloomsburg, PA

Penn State Milton S Hershey Medical Center Program
Hershey, PA

Jefferson Health Medical Education/Jefferson Einstein Philadelphia Hospital Moss Rehab Program
Philadelphia, PA

Temple University Hospital Program
Philadelphia, PA

Sidney Kimmel Medical College at Thomas Jefferson University/TJUH Program
Philadelphia, PA

University of Pennsylvania Health System Program
Philadelphia, PA

UPMC Medical Education Program
Pittsburgh, PA

Wright Center for Graduate Medical Education Program
Scranton, PA

Tower Health Program
Wyomissing, PA

University of Puerto Rico Program
San Juan, PR

VA Caribbean Healthcare System Program
San Juan, PR

HCA Healthcare/Mercer University School of Medicine Program
N Charleston, SC

Vanderbilt University Medical Center Program
Nashville, TN

HCA Healthcare/TriStar Nashville Program
Nashville, TN

University of Texas at Austin Dell Medical School Program
Austin, TX

Baylor University Medical Center Program
Dallas, TX

University of Texas Southwestern Medical Center Program
Dallas, TX

Texas Rehabilitation Hospital of Fort Worth Program
Fort Worth, TX

Baylor College of Medicine Program
Houston, TX

University of Texas Health Science Center at Houston Program
Houston, TX

Texas Tech University Health Sciences Center at Lubbock Program
Lubbock, TX

University of Texas Health Science Center San Antonio Joe and Teresa Lozano Long School of Medicine Program
San Antonio, TX

University of Utah Health Program
Salt Lake City, UT

University of Virginia Medical Center Program
Charlottesville, VA

Eastern Virginia Medical School at Old Dominion University Program
Norfolk, VA

Virginia Commonwealth University Health System Program
Richmond, VA

University of Washington Program
Seattle, WA

Providence Sacred Heart Medical Center Program
Spokane, WA

University of Wisconsin Hospitals and Clinics Program
Madison, WI

Medical College of Wisconsin Affiliated Hospitals Program
Milwaukee, WI

West Virginia University School of Medicine Program
Morgantown, WV

APPENDIX Diii

RESIDENCY PROGRAMS BY STATE NEUROLOGY

APPENDIX Diii

RESIDENCY PROGRAMS BY STATE
NEUROLOGY

Please visit AMA/FREIDA online for detailed and up to date information on programs.
https://freida.ama-assn.org
The following information is provided based on free online resources and program websites.

NEUROLOGY
University of Alabama Medical Center Program
Birmingham, AL

USA Health Program
Mobile, AL

University of Arkansas for Medical Sciences (UAMS) College of Medicine Program
Little Rock, AR

University of Arizona College of Medicine-Phoenix Program
Phoenix, AZ

Barrow Neurological Institute at St Joseph's Hospital and Medical Center Program
Phoenix, AZ

Mayo Clinic College of Medicine and Science (Scottsdale)Program
Scottsdale, AZ

University of Arizona College of Medicine-Tucson Program
Tucson, AZ

Arrowhead Regional Medical Center Program
Colton, CA

Loma Linda University Health Education Consortium Program
Loma Linda, CA
ID: 1800521124

Kaiser Permanente Southern California (Los Angeles) Program
Los Angeles, CA

University of Southern California/Los Angeles General Medical Center (USC/LA General) Program
Los Angeles, CA

UCLA David Geffen School of Medicine/UCLA Medical Center Program
Los Angeles, CA

Cedars-Sinai Medical Center Program
Los Angeles, CA

Riverside University Health System Program
Moreno Valley, CA

University of California (Irvine) Program
Orange, CA

Desert Regional Medical Center Program
Palm Springs, CA

Stanford Health Care-Sponsored Stanford University Program
Palo Alto, CA

Neurology Group Program
Pomona, CA

HCA Healthcare Riverside Program
Riverside, CA

University of California Davis Health Program
Sacramento, CA

University of California (San Diego) Medical Center Program
San Diego, CA

University of California (San Francisco) Program
San Francisco, CA

St Joseph's Medical Center Program
Stockton, CA

HCA Healthcare/Los Robles Regional Medical Center Program
Thousand Oaks, CA

Los Angeles County-Harbor-UCLA Medical Center Program
Torrance, CA

University of Colorado Program
Aurora, CO

HCA Health One/Swedish Medical Center Program
Englewood, CO

University of Connecticut Program
Hartford, CT

Yale-New Haven Medical Center Program
New Haven, CT

MedStar Health/Georgetown University Hospital Program
Washington, DC

George Washington University Program
Washington, DC

Howard University Program
Washington, DC

Florida Atlantic University Charles E Schmidt College of Medicine Program
Boca Raton, FL

Broward Health Program
Deerfield Beach, FL

University of Florida Program
Gainesville, FL

Palmetto General Hospital Program
Hialeah, FL

Larkin Community Hospital Palm Springs Campus Program
Hialeah, FL

Memorial Healthcare System (Hollywood Florida) Program
Hollywood, FL

University of Florida College of Medicine Jacksonville Program
Jacksonville, FL

Mayo Clinic College of Medicine and Science (Jacksonville)Program
Jacksonville, FL

University of Central Florida/HCA Florida Healthcare (Greater Orlando/Osceola) Program
Kissimmee, FL

HCA Florida Healthcare/Westside/Northwest Hospital Program
Margate, FL

Florida International University/Baptist Health Program
Miami, FL

HCA Florida Healthcare Program
Miami, FL

University of Miami/Jackson Health System Program
Miami, FL

Orlando Health Program
Orlando, FL

Larkin Community Hospital Program
South Miami, FL

University of South Florida Morsani Program
Tampa, FL

Cleveland Clinic (Florida) Program
Weston, FL

Emory University School of Medicine Program
Atlanta, GA

Medical College of Georgia Program
Augusta, GA

University of Iowa Hospitals and Clinics Program
Iowa City, IA

Rush University Medical Center Program
Chicago, IL

McGaw Medical Center of Northwestern University Program
Chicago, IL

University of Chicago Program
Chicago, IL

University of Illinois College of Medicine at Chicago Program
Chicago, IL

Loyola University Medical Center Program
Maywood, IL

University of Illinois College of Medicine at Peoria Program
Peoria, IL

Southern Illinois University Program
Springfield, IL

Carle Foundation Hospital Program
Urbana, IL

Indiana University School of Medicine Program
Indianapolis, IN

University of Kansas School of Medicine Program
Kansas City, KS

University of Kentucky College of Medicine Program
Lexington, KY

University of Louisville School of Medicine Program
Louisville, KY

Ochsner Clinic Foundation Program
New Orleans, LA

Louisiana State University School of Medicine Program
New Orleans, LA

Tulane University Program
New Orleans, LA

Louisiana State University (Shreveport) Program
Shreveport, LA

Beth Israel Deaconess Medical Center/Harvard Medical School Program
Boston, MA

Tufts Medical Center Program
Boston, MA

Boston University Medical Center Program
Boston, MA

Mass General Brigham/Brigham and Women's Hospital/Massachusetts General Hospital/Harvard Medical School Program
Boston, MA

UMass Chan Medical School Program
Worcester, MA

Ascension Macomb-Oakland Hospital Program
Worcester, MA

Johns Hopkins University Program
Baltimore, MD

University of Maryland Program
Baltimore, MD

National Capital Consortium Program
Bethesda, MD

Maine Health Program
Portland, ME

University of Michigan Program
Ann Arbor, MI

Henry Ford Health/Henry Ford Hospital Program
Detroit, MI

Detroit Medical Center/Wayne State University Program
Detroit, MI

University of Michigan Health - Sparrow/Michigan State University Program
East Lansing, MI

Corewell Health (Farmington Hills and Royal Oak) Program
Farmington Hills, MI

Garden City Hospital Program
Garden City, MI

Trinity Health Grand Rapids Program
Grand Rapids, MI

Corewell Health-Grand Rapids/Michigan State University Program
Grand Rapids, MI

University of Minnesota Program
Minneapolis, MN

Mayo Clinic College of Medicine and Science (Rochester)Program
Rochester, MN

University of Missouri-Columbia Program
Columbia, MO

University of Missouri-Kansas City School of Medicine Program
Kansas City, MO

SSM Health/Saint Louis University School of Medicine Program
St Louis, MO

Washington University/B-JH/SLCH Consortium Program
St Louis, MO

University of Mississippi Medical Center Program
Jackson, MS

University of North Carolina Hospitals Program
Chapel Hill, NC

Carolinas Medical Center Program
Charlotte, NC

Duke University Hospital Program
Durham, NC
ID: 1803621085

ECU Health Medical Center Program
Greenville, NC

Wake Forest University Baptist Medical Center Program
Winston-Salem, NC

University of North Dakota School of Medicine and Health Sciences Program
Fargo, ND

Creighton University School of Medicine (Omaha) Program
Omaha, NE

University of Nebraska Medical Center College of Medicine Program
Omaha, NE

Dartmouth-Hitchcock/Mary Hitchcock Memorial Hospital Program
Lebanon, NH

Cooper Medical School of Rowan University/Cooper University Hospital Program
Camden, NJ

JFK Medical Center Program
Edison, NJ

Rutgers Health/Robert Wood Johnson Medical School Program
New Brunswick, NJ

Rutgers Health/New Jersey Medical School Program
Newark, NJ

University of New Mexico School of Medicine Program
Albuquerque, NM

OPTI West/Valley Hospital Medical Center Program
Las Vegas, NV

HCA Healthcare Sunrise Health GME/Southern Hills Program
Las Vegas, NV

Albany Medical Center Program
Albany, NY

Montefiore Medical Center/Albert Einstein College of Medicine Program
Bronx, NY

SUNY Downstate Health Sciences University/One Brooklyn Health System Program
Brooklyn, NY

SUNY Downstate Health Sciences University Program
Brooklyn, NY

University at Buffalo Program
Buffalo, NY

Zucker School of Medicine at Hofstra/Northwell Program
Manhasset, NY

Garnet Health Medical Center Program
Middletown, NY

NYU Long Island School of Medicine Program
Mineola, NY

Icahn School of Medicine at Mount Sinai/West Program
New York, NY

New York Presbyterian Hospital (Cornell Campus) Program
New York, NY

Icahn School of Medicine at Mount Sinai/Mount Sinai Hospital Program
New York, NY

NYU Grossman School of Medicine Program
New York, NY

New York Presbyterian Hospital (Columbia Campus) Program
New York, NY

Nuvance Health Program
Poughkeepsie, NY

University of Rochester Program
Rochester, NY

Zucker School of Medicine at Hofstra/Northwell at Staten Island University Hospital Program
Staten Island, NY

Stony Brook Medicine/University Hospital Program
Stony Brook, NY

SUNY Upstate Medical University Program
Syracuse, NY

Westchester Medical Center Program
Valhalla, NY

University of Cincinnati Medical Center/College of Medicine Program
Cincinnati, OH

Case Western Reserve University/University Hospitals Cleveland Medical Center Program
Cleveland, OH

Cleveland Clinic Foundation Program
Cleveland, OH

Ohio State University Hospital Program
Columbus, OH

Wright State University Boonshoft School of Medicine Program
Dayton, OH

Kettering Health Network Program
Dayton, OH

University of Toledo Program
Toledo, OH

Mercy St Vincent Medical Center Program
Toledo, OH

University of Oklahoma Health Sciences Center Program
Oklahoma City, OK

Oregon Health & Science University (OHSU Health) Program
Portland, OR

Lehigh Valley Health Network Program
Allentown, PA

Geisinger Health System (Danville) Program
Danville, PA

St Luke's Hospital-Anderson Campus Program
Easton, PA

UPMC Medical Education (Erie) Program
Erie, PA

Penn State Milton S Hershey Medical Center Program
Hershey, PA

Temple University Hospital Program
Philadelphia, PA

Sidney Kimmel Medical College at Thomas Jefferson University/TJUH Program
Philadelphia, PA

University of Pennsylvania Health System Program
Philadelphia, PA

Jefferson Health Medical Education/Jefferson Einstein Philadelphia Hospital Program
Philadelphia, PA

UPMC Medical Education (Pittsburgh) Program
Pittsburgh, PA

Allegheny Health Network Medical Education Consortium (AGH)Program
Pittsburgh, PA

Tower Health Program
West Reading, PA

Geisinger Health System Program (Wilkes-Barre)
Wilkes-Barre, PA

University of Puerto Rico Program
San Juan, PR

Brown University Program
Providence, RI

Medical University of South Carolina Program
Charleston, SC

Prisma Health/University of South Carolina School of Medicine Columbia (Columbia) Program
Columbia, SC

Prisma Health/University of South Carolina School of Medicine Columbia (Greer) Program
Greer, SC

University of South Dakota School of Medicine Program
Sioux Falls, SD

University of Tennessee College of Medicine-Chattanooga Program
Chattanooga, TN

University of Tennessee Graduate School of Medicine Program

University of Tennessee Program
Memphis, TN

Vanderbilt University Medical Center Program
Nashville, TN

HCA Healthcare/TriStar Nashville/Skyline Medical Center Program
Nashville, TN

University of Texas at Austin Dell Medical School/Ascension Seton Medical Center Program
Austin, TX

University of Texas at Austin Dell Medical School/Dell Seton Medical Center Program
Austin, TX

University of Texas Southwestern Medical Center Program
Dallas, TX

Texas Tech University HSC El Paso Program
El Paso, TX

University of Texas Medical Branch Hospitals Program
Galveston, TX

University of Texas Rio Grande Valley Program
Harlingen, TX

Methodist Hospital (Houston) Program
Houston, TX

Baylor College of Medicine Program
Houston, TX

University of Texas Health Science Center at Houston Program
Houston, TX

San Antonio Uniformed Services Health Education Consortium Program
JBSA Ft Sam Houston, TX

Texas Tech University Health Sciences Center at Lubbock Program
Lubbock, TX

University of Texas Health Science Center San Antonio Joe and Teresa Lozano Long School of Medicine Program

San Antonio, TX

Texas A&M College of Medicine-Scott and White Medical Center (Temple) Program
Temple, TX

University of Texas Health Science Center at Tyler Program
Tyler, TX

University of Utah Health Program
Salt Lake City, UT

University of Virginia Medical Center Program
Charlottesville, VA

Virginia Commonwealth University Health System Program
Richmond, VA

Carilion Clinic-Virginia Tech Carilion School of Medicine Program
Roanoke, VA

University of Vermont Medical Center Program
Burlington, VT

University of Washington Program
Seattle, WA

Madigan Army Medical Center Program
Tacoma, WA

University of Wisconsin Hospitals and Clinics Program
Madison, WI

Medical College of Wisconsin Affiliated Hospitals Program
Milwaukee, WI

Charleston Area Medical Center Program
Charleston, WV

Marshall University School of Medicine Program
Huntington, WV

West Virginia University Program
Morgantown, WV

GLOSSARY

AAMC – Association of American Medical Colleges

ABMS – American Board of Medical Specialties

ACGME – Accreditation Council on Graduate Medical Education

AMA – American Medical Association

ECFMG – Educational Commission on Foreign Medical Graduates

ERAS – Electronic Residency Application Service

FMG – Foreign Medical Graduate

FSMB – Federation of State Medical Boards

GME – Graduate Medical Education

IMG – International Medical graduate

IWA – Interactive Web Application

MSPE – Medical Student Performance Evaluation

NBME – National Board of Medical Examiners

NRMP – National Residency Matching Program

OASIS – Online Applicant Status and Information System

PTAL – Post-graduate Training Authorization Letter

SEVIS – Student and Exchange Visitor Information System

SOAP – Supplemental Offer and Acceptance Program

USCIS – U.S. Citizenship and Immigration Services

USMLE – U.S. Medical Licensing Examination

USMLE CK – Clinical Knowledge

USMLE CS – Clinical Skills

INDEX

AAFP, 13
AAMC, 10, 17
AAPM&R, 13
ACGME, 8
ADTS, 29
Advanced programs, 15
AMA, 13
American Medical Association (AMA), 9
Categorical programs, 14
Clerkship performance, 31
Dependent visa, 64
ECFMG, 6
ECFMG certificate, 8
ERAS, 10
ERAS application, 10
ERAS documents, 19
ERAS season, 10
Family Medicine, 14
FREIDA, 9
H1B visa program, 64
Internal Medicine, 14
International medical graduates (IMGs), 6
J-1 Visa program, 63
Medical school Performance, 31
MSPE, 20, 33
National Residency Match Program NRMP, 11
NBME Mock, 12
Neurology, 14
NRMP, 50
NRMP MATCH, 54
Pediatrics, 14
Physical Medicine and Rehabilitation, 14
Radiology, 14
residency application, 2
Residency positions, 3

residency process, 1
residency training, 2
S.O.A.P, 58
the letters of recommendations, 2
US Graduates, 6
US Health care system, 1
USMLE, 1
USMLE performance, 5
USMLE resources, 7
Visa Requirements, 62

NOTES

NOTES

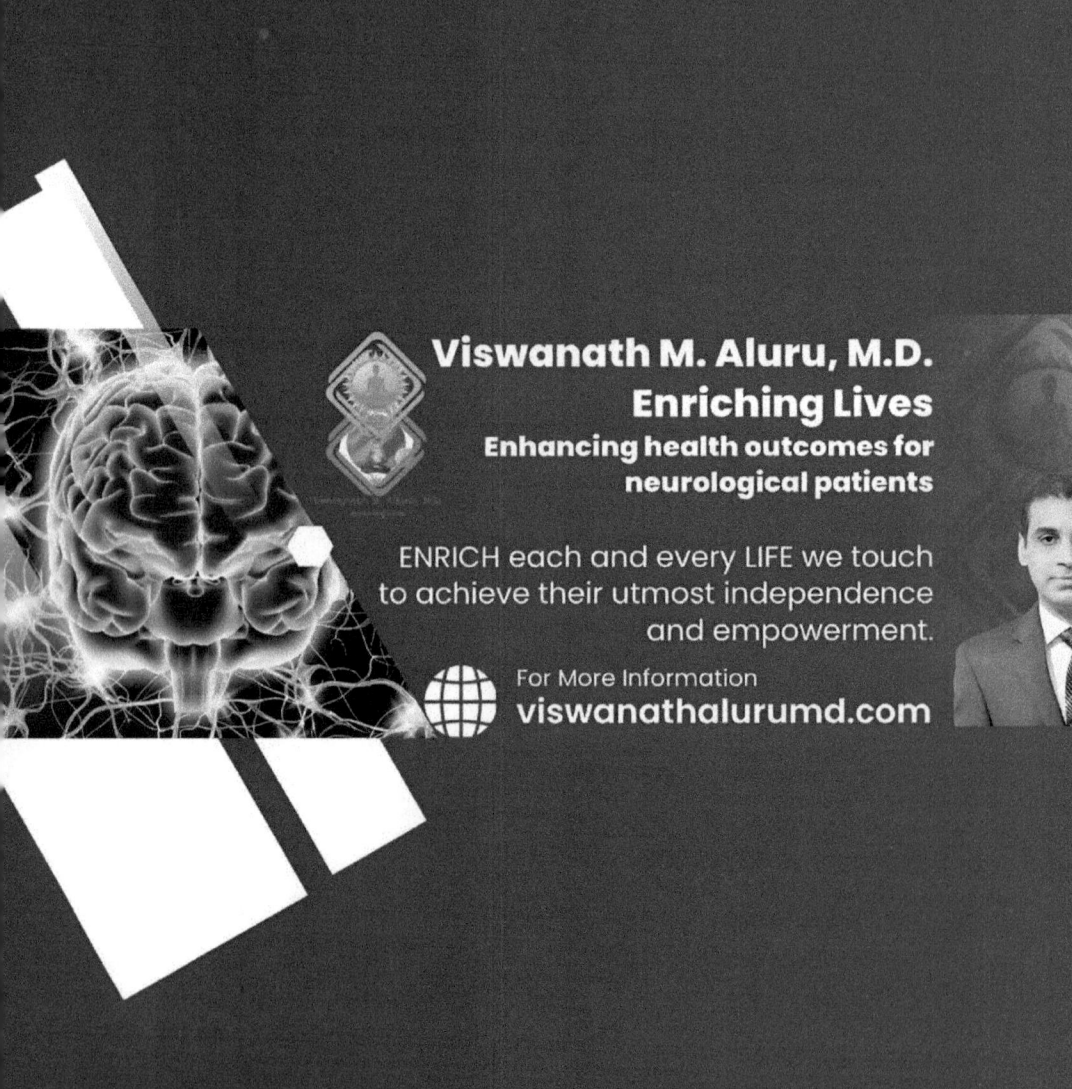

www.ingramcontent.com/pod-product-compliance
Lightning Source LLC
Chambersburg PA
CBHW071714090426
42738CB00009B/1776